THE YOGA OF
BREATH

BOOKS AND AUDIO BY
RICHARD ROSEN

BOOKS

Original Yoga
Pranayama beyond the Fundamentals
The Yoga of Breath

AUDIO

The Practice of Pranayama

THE YOGA OF
BREATH

*A Step-by-Step Guide
to Pranayama*

RICHARD ROSEN

Foreword by Rodney Yee
Illustrations by Kim Fraley

SHAMBHALA
Boston & London
2002

To: Laura and Taleen

We know that it is the search that gives meaning to any find and that one often has to travel a long way in order to arrive at what is near.

—José Saramago, *All the Names*

Shambhala Publications, Inc.
Horticultural Hall
300 Massachusetts Avenue
Boston, Massachusetts 02115
www.shambhala.com

©2002 by Richard Rosen

16 15 14 13 12 11 10

Printed in the United States of America

⊗ This edition is printed on acid-free paper that meets the American National Standards Institute Z39.48 Standard.

♻ This book is printed on 30% postconsumer recycled paper. For more information please visit www.shambhala.com.

Distributed in the United States by Penguin Random House LLC and in Canada by Random House of Canada Ltd

Interior design and composition: Greta D. Sibley & Associates

Library of Congress Cataloging-in-Publication Data
Rosen, Richard.
The yoga of breath: a step-by-step guide to Pranayama / Richard Rosen; foreword by Rodney Yee.
p. cm.
Includes bibliographical references and index.
ISBN 978-1-57062-889-4
1. Breathing exercises. 2. Yoga, Hatha. I. Title.
RA781.7.R665 2002
613.7'046—dc21
2002017657

CONTENTS

FOREWORD

A COOL BREEZE on the sweat of your brow on a hot summer day—that's how I feel every morning when I take my first sips of conscious air. At this point it takes very little time for this feeling to drop me into a place of delight and wonder. When did these observations of my breath become such a consoling friend? For as I tell my students and friends, it is my pranayama practice, not my asana or meditation practice, that is most precious to me. Every day for the last fifteen years, I have started my day with pranayama. I reserve time for my pranayama practice in the morning no matter where I am or what I'm doing—whether I'm on an airplane or my kids are running in and out of the room—to completely detach from my surroundings and go inward. I look forward to it more than I look forward to a good night's sleep. It is both a great solace and a wonderful way to understand who I am today before I enter into relationship with the outside world.

Can I recall the first time I folded a bolster and lay down under the meticulous instructions of my yoga teacher? I was wondering why the teacher was being so fussy. I was wondering why the blanket had to be so neat and my body so symmetrical. I felt as if I were being called to some secret order and blindfolded as I was being led to the sanctuary. And when I actually began going into the realm of the breath, my mind didn't have the steadiness that was required to notice any of the subtleties of my breath. But I still had miraculous effects now and again, which were enough to lead me on. I remember ending up in some states of mind of ethereal peace and states of my body of infinite space that seemed as if they were from a different galaxy.

Then one day my pranayama teacher looked me in the eyes and said—not with sternness but in a matter-of-fact tone—"Either take this practice on daily or let it go." So at that point I began my daily practice of pranayama, due partly to my trust of my teacher and partly to a personal intuition that told me this was a vital practice for me. With each ensuing year my fondness of the practice has deepened because it is so enticing to be led by my breath instead of my mind, for at least part of my day. And because I found pranayama so useful for my own daily life, I began to teach it weekly at my studio, wanting to share this practice with my students and colleagues.

All that time, right next to me, day after day, my friend Richard Rosen was also wrestling with this practice. During those early days we were commuting back and forth to yoga class, then having lunch together and discussing asana, pranayama, and everything else under the sun. For both of us the asana practice was extremely difficult. We were both very tight and emotionally frustrated with this tightness. We practiced two or three times a week together, devising ways to penetrate our thick, tight, immovable bodies. We stepped on each other, pushed each other, and joked about our difficulties. Richard was as much in love with the practice as I was, and just as tenacious. However, our guylike approach to the asanas was beginning to crack from our constant work trying to uncover the subtleties of our breath. We would lie down next to each other—one of us invariably falling asleep—trying to adhere our minds to our breath. And although I could never really know all the feelings, thoughts, and physical sensations that he experienced, somehow I knew we were both absorbing the same divine fragrance. After pranayama something about the changes in his eyes and his skin were the signs that we had ended up in a similar place, although we had traveled through different terrain to get there. (Sometimes I can go into a room full of yogis and know who in that room is practicing pranayama because of their relaxed tone of voice and the light inside their eyes.)

The practice of yoga promises liberation, and Richard has been unrelenting in his quest for freedom. He has spent many, many hours both in search of and inside his breath. The yogis say that the breath is the ruler of the mind and body. But it takes years to let the mind relinquish its illusion of control. By letting the mind play games with the breath, day after day, year after year, there is a point when the mind gives up its folly. Then we can allow the mind to be immersed in the ocean of prana. Richard has looked deeply into his own psyche, his body, and his breath to try to solve the riddle of his imprisonment, and even as he moves in this direction, he generously lends his help to both his colleagues and his students.

Looking back on our friendship, Richard was the best yoga buddy I could have had. He was always willing to experiment, trying things that I came up with and being innovative himself with props and postures to wake up the consciousness in different parts of our bodies and minds. And even though many times we took very different paths, he was always open to seeing my point of view. He has also been a steady source of inspiration and courage for me. He was always able to stand firm in his beliefs and go his own way, even when it was difficult. And whenever he had problems with other people, he would be much more likely to find out why he was bothered and what internal changes he needed to make. I always found him to be harder on himself than on anybody else. So he has inspired me to take responsibility for my actions and my inadequacies. Now as I look into Richard's eyes, once again I find companionship. He feels like both a friend and a father, someone who understands my history and continues to walk beside me.

For many years I've seen Richard evolve as a teacher. He has taught full-time for fifteen years and has a loyal following of students whom he guides with great care and concern. And he has worked arduously to hone his skills as a teacher so that he can share his rich knowledge of yoga. He is one of the most well read yoga instructors in the United States, and I often go to him with questions about the yoga texts and the history of yoga. And because Richard has struggled deeply himself, he has great compassion for students who are also grappling with these practices.

Both Richard and I know how hard it is to teach an ongoing pranayama class. Many people say they want to learn about the breath, but few are patient enough to uncover the benefits. We both have tried very hard to find ways to entice people to take on this practice because we know how valuable pranayama is for us as human beings. And I believe that his years of dedication and experimentation have enabled Richard to crack the code, allowing him to inspire his students to maintain a continuing pranayama practice. So I'm very happy that this book gives Richard the opportunity to get this wealth of knowledge down in writing for the benefit of us all.

For the very beginner Richard offers a methodical way to see and understand the breath. For people who have an asana practice but not a pranayama practice, Richard will intrigue you and invite you into the infinite mystery of the breath. For those learning how to teach pranayama, this book is a great manual to follow week by week. It provides a very comprehensive yogic view of the breath that I know I find helpful. Whereas some of my recollections of my pranayama practices are a bunch of half-heard babbling going in and out of a dream, Richard used his study of classical yoga literature and his own experiences, which he documented in his journals, to thoroughly map the terrain through which he has breathed. There is still a lot of basic knowledge about pranayama that I myself have not yet acquired, so I personally look forward to using his book to round out my knowledge and to deepen my pranayama practice through the simple, profound exercises Richard has laid out for us.

Sometimes I picture the two of us in old age, Richard and me, not in rocking chairs, but sitting on the ground in lotus, listening to the wheezing of our breath and laughing at the folly of our lives. Thanks, Richard.

—Rodney Yee

ACKNOWLEDGMENTS

THERE ARE a lot of people I want to acknowledge for helping me with this book. First off, there are my editors at Shambhala Publications, Dan Spinella and Beth Frankl, who have managed to make me look like a much better writer than I actually am.

Thanks too to Nina Zolotow for helping Rodney put together his wonderful foreword to this guide.

The drawings that grace this guide are the result of a collaboration among three people: Paulette Traverso, my unofficial art director; Vickie Russell Bell, my model; and Kim Fraley, illustrator extraordinaire. Thanks to you all.

I can't forget my good friend and mentor Georg Feuerstein, who's taught me everything I need to know about the yoga tradition and more. I had the opportunity to lead regular pranayama courses at the Yoga Room in Berkeley for a decade. Thanks to Donald Moyer, the school's director and guiding light.

I owe an enormous debt of gratitude to B. K. S. Iyengar, a truly monumental figure in contemporary yoga. Without his teaching, this guide would simply not exist.

And finally I want to tip my hat to my pranayama teachers over the last twenty years, Manouso Manos, Arthur Kilmurray, and Ramanand Patel. Pretty much everything of any value I have to offer here I've learned from them, while all the mistakes are mine alone.

Colloquy of the Vital Breaths

Prana-Samvada

NOW ONCE UPON A TIME, Tongue, Eye, Ear, Mind, and Breath were arguing about who was the best among them, who was the most important to the life of the body. They appealed to their father, Prajapati, the Lord-of-Creation, for his opinion. "Sir," they cried, "who is the best of us?" The wise Prajapati suggested a simple way to settle the dispute: "He by whose departure the body seems worse than worst, he is the best of you."

First Tongue left for a year, and when he came back he asked, "How have you been able to live without me?" And the others replied, "Like mute people, not speaking," yet they were able to see, hear, think, and breathe just fine. So Tongue was not the best.

Next Eye left for a year, and when he came back he asked, "How have you been able to live without me?" And the others replied, "Like blind people, not seeing," yet they were able to talk, hear, think, and breathe just fine. So Eye was not the best.

Then Ear left for a year, and when he came back he asked, "How have you been able to live without me?" And the others replied, "Like deaf people, not hearing," yet they were able to talk, see, think, and breathe just fine. So Ear was not the best.

Off went Mind for a year, and when he came back he asked, "How have you been able to live without me?" And the others replied, "Like children whose mind is not yet formed," yet they were able to talk, see, hear, and breathe just fine. So Mind was not the best.

Finally, as Breath got ready to go, she ripped at the other breaths, "as a horse, going to start, might tear up the pegs to which he is tethered." The others realized immediately that they couldn't live without Breath. "Madam," they cried, "thou art the best among us. Do not depart from us!"

And so, the parable concludes, people don't call these five the Vital Tongues, the Vital Eyes, the Vital Ears, or the Vital Minds, but the Vital Breaths (prana), "for the vital breath is all these."

> —Chandogya-Upanishad, in *The Thirteen Principal Upanishads*, quoted dialogue translated by Robert Ernest Hume

THE YOGA OF
BREATH

Lions, Elephants, Tigers

Just as lions, elephants and tigers are gradually controlled, so the prana is controlled through practice. Otherwise the practitioner is destroyed. By proper practice of pranayama, all diseases are eradicated. Through improper practice, all diseases can arise.

—Svatmarama, *Hatha-Yoga-Pradipika*

SIXTEEN YEARS AGO my wife and I went on a five-month trip through China, Tibet, Nepal, and India. For the whole time we acted as our own travel agents, porters, and—for a couple of truly awful days after we ate something we shouldn't have—doctors.

We naturally brought along a couple of guidebooks, familiar companions to most travelers. They included all kinds of useful information: background on the countries' history and culture, maps of the territory and its cities, tips on how to get around in buses and trains, what kinds of things to bring along and what to wear, what to see when you get to your destination, and where to stay and eat—and what to avoid. Everything, in other words, that the bewildered tourist needs to know to get from point A to point B and back home with the minimum amount of fuss.

I'm mentioning all this because these guides are very similar, I believe, to other kinds of guides many of us have run across in our lives, written by spiritual travelers. I don't suppose we ordinarily think of yogis as being travelers. We picture these folks holed up in their caves or monasteries on isolated mountaintops, spending their days hunkered in the same spot, deep in meditation or some other otherworldly pursuit. But the yogis are travelers, who over the centuries have marched off on adventures into the vast and largely uncharted realm of human consciousness, what I call the country of the Self.

A trip into this country isn't for the fainthearted. As you probably already know, it's difficult to get started, the way is checkered
with hidden pitfalls and alluring detours, and there's never any guarantee that you'll get back with all your luggage or in good health.
But a few yogis do return in one piece. Sometimes they want to
share with us what they've seen and heard and felt and learned, just
in case we want to visit the country of the Self, too, even though we
may wonder what we'll do about child care and the mortgage. Their
guides make the journey seem less daunting, more accessible to
those of us who live in the everyday world. They tell us what to expect
and obstacles to avoid, the safest trails to follow, how to equip ourselves, and what to do and where to go when we get there.

There's one area in which my analogy between the two kinds of
guidebooks isn't so tidy. We like the writing in our guides to be clear
and straightforward. The last thing we want is confusing or vague
directions when we're stuck in the middle of nowhere. But often,
because their experiences in the country of the Self are so out of the
ordinary, the yogis can't find the right words to describe them ade-
quately. So many of their guides, both old and new, aren't written
as succinctly as we'd like, and we have to work a bit harder to understand their directions. Sometimes they resort to poetry, as they did
in the ancient Upanishads, the once-secret writings that form the basis
of the Vedanta philosophy, or in the famous Bhagavad-Gita, the
Lord's Song, often called the New Testament of Hinduism.

Other times the yogis pen cryptic aphorisms, called sutras, that
afford only the barest hints of their journey. Without an added commentary, either oral or written, by another expert spiritual traveler,
these sutra guides can be mystifying, if not downright opaque. Such
is the case with the first systematic guide to yoga, the Yoga-Sutra,
compiled by the sage Patanjali about eighteen hundred years ago.
A sutra is literally a "thread" or "string." This Sanskrit word is related
to the English sew and suture. By itself it relays only the barest
thread of information. Some scholars argue that a sutra guide is
really a mnemonic device, a means for the student to string together
and organize her teacher's more extensive instructions about the
journey. (We'll look more closely at the Yoga-Sutra and its teaching
on pranayama in chapter 2.)

You may or may not already have some experience with yoga. If you do, it's probably mostly with the yoga postures, or asanas. Though pranayama often takes a backseat to a vigorous program of asanas, traditionally it's the other way round. In the schools that teach both practices—and not all schools of yoga do—asana is primarily a preparation for the more advanced and time-consuming practice of pranayama. Pranayama is usually translated as "breath control," and while this is a convenient and to a certain extent accurate way to understand pranayama, it doesn't tell the whole story.

Just as there are many different schools of yoga, so also are there different approaches to pranayama. The one we'll take here follows the pioneering work of B. K. S. Iyengar, who has, over the last fifty or so years, developed a rigorous brand of practice that, while it honors the long yoga tradition, is uniquely his own. His approach can be characterized as slow and steady, which is the best way to go whenever learning something new. It emphasizes how things are done and not so much what is done. I call it the lions, elephants, and tigers approach, a reference to a verse quoted above from the Hatha-Yoga-Pradipika.

I had my first taste of pranayama in 1983, in a twelve-week introductory course at the Iyengar Yoga Institute in San Francisco. I'd like to say that those long-ago twelve weeks transformed my life completely, that through pranayama I had deep insights and luminous visions that revealed the essence of my authentic self. I'd like to say that . . . but I can't, because it wouldn't be true. The truth is, I had a pretty awful time.

The trouble started immediately in the first class. Since I was studying at an Iyengar school, I was required, as a beginner, to recline for my practice on folded blankets (we'll talk about why reclining is important in chapter 13). Then the teacher asked the class to pay close attention to the movement of our inhales and exhales, to slow them down as much as possible, and to fill every nook and cranny of our lungs with air.

But when I tried to take my first slow, full inhale, it seemed as if I had a ton of bricks stacked on my chest, squashing my lungs. I noticed, too, that my brain ballooned dangerously, threatening to burst out through the top of my skull. The exhale wasn't promising either. My throat clenched tight like a fist, and by the time the out-going breath shuddered to an end, I was gasping for the next inhale like a fish out of water. My pranayama career was off to a slow start, and then—as a defeated presidential candidate once said of his campaign—things went downhill from there.

In a few weeks I developed a knot of tension at the bottom of my sternum, where the diaphragm attaches to the bone. If I pushed on it with my thumb, the pain made me want to cry. I never did, but I probably should have. After every class I felt confused, anxious, irritable. I got headaches.

My pranayama teacher was sympathetic. He tried everything he could think of to help me: different kinds of blanket supports, sand-bags pressing down on my thighs and forehead, various exercises to stretch my chest and belly and quiet my brain to prepare for breathing. Still I suffered.

I huffed and puffed my way through the intermediate and advanced courses with no improvement. Then I continued on my own after the third course ended, despite my travail. Bright and early every morning, I diligently worked on my pranayama for an hour. I refused to give up and take things lying down (figuratively speaking, that is). I experimented on myself, inventing fantastically shaped reclining supports constructed out of blankets and towels, tennis balls, wood planks, two-pound lead fishing weights, broom-sticks, metal folding chairs, even heavy cardboard packing tubes. For a while I practiced a few times each week in my bathtub, up to my neck in warm water.

There were days when my breathing seemed to turn a corner, and I thought that maybe I was on the verge of a breakthrough. Then inevitably I did an abrupt about-face and unimproved back to where I was before. I took some solace in Mr. Iyengar's dictum that prac-tice waxes and wanes like the moon. Mine sure did, though it hardly ever waxed, and mostly it waned.

Finally, after about four or five years, I had a breathing experi-ence that really did profoundly affect my life. I was lying on my blankets with my ton of bricks in place on my chest, and my teacher gave the class a simple instruction. "On the next inhalation," he said, "allow your spine to lift off the support and up into your back." By this time I was a well-trained Iyengar student, and that sounded like a reasonable enough request, so I did it . . . and whoosh, my chest exploded, and this flood of air effortlessly surged into my lungs. I was so surprised that my closed eyes popped wide open and my jaw dropped onto my chest. It was such a jolt, in fact, that I actually stopped breathing. I felt light as a feather, as if I were about to float up and bump into the ceiling, and yet at the same time as deeply rooted to the earth as a tree. I suddenly understood in my heart of hearts what it meant to be totally alive. I wondered, Is this what my very first breath was like?

I quickly tried to re-create the sensation on my next inhale and the next after that and the next after that. I prayed each time for another miracle, but nothing happened. My ton of bricks, momentarily hoisted off my chest, was lowered down again.

But strangely I wasn't at all discouraged. Though it lasted for only a few seconds, that single inhalation had jolted me awake and revealed the limitless possibilities of pranayama. I had a picture of this long extension cord emerging from my spine and plugged into the Source of everything. Somewhere inside me the switch was OFF, but I knew that it was just a matter of time before I figured out how to flip it to ON.

The instruction in this guide will prepare you for and then take you through your first year or so of the practice. I've divided it into four parts. Four is a highly significant number in the yoga and Hindu traditions. It represents the "fulfillment of manifestations in all the spheres of existence, the four stages that may be found in every form of development, of life."[1] So four conveys the "idea of total, or totality. . . . Anything complete and self-contained is conceived as possessing all of its four 'quarters' (pada). It is thus established firmly on its 'four legs.'"[2] Many of the old yoga guides, such as the Yoga-Sutra and the Hatha-Yoga-Pradipika, have four chapters, which indicates that they're complete and self-contained teachings. There are also four traditional stages (avastha) in the development of spiritual exercise, whether considering yoga as a whole or just one of its individual practices, like pranayama. Each of these stages is marked by (what seem to us) strange experiences and the acquisition of even stranger powers.

We're told, for example, that in the beginning stage (arambha-avastha), the aspirant's body becomes "lustrous and brilliant with a divine smell and diseaseless."[3] The second stage is called the stage of the vessel (ghata-avastha) because the aspirant's consciousness is filled with sounds or voices (nada), much as a vessel or pot is filled with water. In the third stage, the stage of accumulation (parichaya-avastha), the aspirant's spiritual power continues to increase or heap up (parichaya) as she "enters the place of total perfection,"[4] where she realizes the end of pain, old age, disease, hunger, and sleep. Finally, in the aptly named stage of maturity or consummation (nishpatti-avastha), the aspirant "drinks the waters of immortality."[5]

While these descriptions of signs and powers suggest the limitless spiritual potential of yoga, they're more than likely out of our reach as beginners in pranayama. I like to think about the four stages in the framework of what I call the four Cs. They serve as a kind of map by which we can chart our journey and check our natural impulse to travel too fast and maybe miss important stops along the way.

Stage 1: clarification (from clarus, "clear, bright"). Here we shine a light on the territory to be explored, things you need to know before you take off into the country of the Self, such as traditional teachings about prana and pranayama, common obstacles encountered by beginning breathers, and useful practice aids, props, and tips.

I'll also invite you to keep a record of your travels in a pranayama journal. One of the main requirements for the students in my eight-week pranayama intensives is that they write a daily account of their practice. To be honest, not everyone enjoys writing in these journals, judging by some of the responses I get. But in general the journal is well received—at least it's preferable to a final essay—and I believe that it's a useful reference point over the long haul.

Stage 2: cooperation (from co-, "with," and opus, "work"). Next we'll begin to survey our physical body and our everyday breath. This will help us put together a kind of physical and psychological profile of ourselves as a breather. The funny thing about traveling in the country of the Self is that, in addition to knowing something about where we're going, we also need to know something about who is going. In this enterprise we'll enlist the help of a new traveling companion, who comes free with this book, the Witness.

Stage 3: comprehension (from com-, "with," and prehendere, "to seize, grasp"). As I mentioned above, asana is traditionally a preparation for pranayama, and so at this stage we'll learn a few simple postures that will get us ready to breathe.

Most approaches to pranayama set the beginning breather up immediately in a sitting position. But in the lions, elephants, and tigers approach, in order to better comprehend or grasp the breath, the early weeks and months of the practice are done while reclining, with the torso and occasionally the legs supported on a prop, usually a folded blanket. We'll also learn how to make the transition from reclining to sitting, and three basic sitting postures.

Stage 4: completion (from com-, "with," and plenus, "full"). Finally we'll turn to two traditional pranayama breaths, the Conqueror (ujjayi) and Against-the-Grain (viloma), supplemented with a few elementary pranayama tools or techniques. Although I call this last stage completion, remember that the journey into the country of the Self never really comes to an end. Every fourth stage is also the first of an entirely new and exciting voyage.

Before we finish this introduction, there are three questions that might be relevant to ask:

Are you sure I even need pranayama? I mean, I'm busy enough now as it is. Why do I need another practice? The answer to the first part of this question is a definite "It all depends." If you're already practicing asana, and using it primarily as a means of physical exercise or stress reduction, you may feel that you're investing all the time you want to in yoga. That's fine. Asana is a great way to get strong and flexible. You should know, however, that pranayama also has a number of health benefits (which I'll talk about in chapter 2) and potentially could make your asana practice even more effective. But if you're applying yourself seriously to yoga as a spiritual exercise, in the quest to realize your authentic self, then the answer to your question is an unqualified yes. Pranayama has been an essential ingredient of yoga for at least two thousand years. I like to think of asana and pranayama and the other traditional limbs of yoga practice, like the behavioral prescripts and meditation, as the strings on my guitar. Take one or two away, and the music just doesn't sound right.

Of course, the only way to know for sure if you need pranayama is to try the practice for yourself. Enter into the work with an open mind and make a commitment to practice wholeheartedly for at least a year. At the end of the allotted time, ask yourself: Does pranayama do what it's advertised to do? Is my overall yoga practice—and my life—enhanced by this work? Then decide for yourself whether to continue along the road.

Can I really learn pranayama—or any yoga practice, for that matter—from a book? Obviously I believe, and so do lots of other writers, that the answer to this question is yes, up to a point. In the old days the guides provided only the bare bones of the practice, which then was always fleshed out with the oral instructions of a living master. Without the support and insight of a spiritual expert, the book was virtually useless.

This guide, however, is meant to provide you with both a theoretical and practical basis of pranayama. Ultimately, though, to develop and complete your practice beyond the beginning stages, you'll have to get the personal help of a qualified teacher. One of the first things they told me in yoga school is to teach only what you know. I've tried to apply this rule in this guide.

I've heard that pranayama is dangerous. Is that true? The beginning practices I'm giving you are safe and sane, tested in the laboratory of my pranayama classes over many years. If you follow my advice patiently and with awareness, you should be fine. It's really not hard to begin pranayama, and once begun, neither is it hard to maintain a basic daily routine.

The material in this guide is arranged sequentially; in other words, you're supposed to start with chapter 1 and end with chapter 20, and not leave out anything in between. If you're like me, though, you're probably rarin' to go and thinking that you can easily skip a chapter here and there in Part One, and dive right into the good stuff in Part Two. But I urge you to take a nice, deep breath, pacify your understandable enthusiasm, and plow your way through the first six chapters. This reading is like the foundation of a house you're about to build: the information in Part One will anchor you firmly in the ground and keep your practice from tipping over in a strong wind.

It's just as important that you take your time and methodically work through Part Two. Make sure you've really understood and fully explored each exercise before you move on to the next. You might even want to do what travelers often do and return to places you've already visited for another look. Think of this stage of your pranayama journey as a leisurely, open-ended tour rather than a race to the finish line. There are lots of interesting things to see and do along the way, and if you're in a hurry, you'll almost surely miss some of the best sights.

This isn't, of course, the only pranayama guidebook in the world. I grew up in pranayama reading B. K. S. Iyengar's *Light on Pranayama*. My weathered copy is, as I type this, in its permanent place on my desk shelf just to my right, within easy reach. What I'm offering here is nothing more than a humble supplement to this classic text. By the same token, the lions, elephants, and tigers approach isn't the only way to go. There are any number of yoga teachers who can make an excellent case for taking a different route. But once you commit yourself to the practice outlined here, then I believe it's best to stick with it exclusively for a while and not introduce any outside elements. When you have some experience with the practice, after a year or so, then it's OK—in fact, I encourage you—to experiment with other possibilities.

PART ONE

Clarification

CHAPTER 1

The Yoga of Breathing

All life is yoga.

—Sri Aurobindo,
The Synthesis of Yoga

Yoga

The classical or literary language of India is Sanskrit. The word itself means "well or completely formed, perfected." Sanskrit is indeed a beautiful and highly evocative language. Many of its words remind me of a Russian doll, which opens up to reveal a smaller doll inside, and which in its turn opens to reveal an even smaller doll, and so on and on until the littlest doll is exposed. Even though I don't know the language well, I can find my way around in a Sanskrit-English dictionary. I like to look up words in the yoga lexicon and pull them apart to see what's inside. This often gives me new insights into my practice. We'll be unraveling Sanskrit words as we go through this guide. Your practice will be enriched by the hidden meanings in this perfect language.

Let's start with a word that may already be familiar to you—the Sanskrit verb *yuj*, which means to "yoke" or "harness." It's a relic of an age, many thousands of years ago, when Indian warriors rode into battle in chariots. These wagons typically carried an archer and his driver or charioteer and were drawn by two horses, which had the reputation of being rather ferocious. "At his deep neigh," sings one old hymn about the cry of a warhorse, "like the thunder of heaven / the foemen tremble in fear." It was the charioteer's task to hitch these barely tamed beasts to the chariot, no small feat in the days before the invention of the yoke. He needed both extraordinary bravery and skill, and as a consequence, his position was highly esteemed.

In the everyday language, yuj assumed the sense of "unite, connect, add, bring together," as well as—since the occupation of yoking or harnessing implied that the charioteer had learned a particular technique that got the chariot up and running—"make ready, prepare, set to work, employ, apply." Two notions, then, of a desired end and its means are conveyed by the verb yuj and its several derivatives, including the masculine noun yoga.

The practice of yoga is very old. There were surely contemporaries of our charioteer who were engaged in some form of yoga, though it probably didn't exactly resemble what we call yoga today. In general, yoga has four goals:

1. Regeneration or health, and the end of suffering
2. Skillful action
3. Integration or self-knowledge
4. Liberation

In much of the sacred literature of India, liberation (moksha) is explained as the yoking or joining of the embodied soul (jiva-atman) to the Great Self (parama-atman). Both yoke and join, by the way, are cognate with yuj and yoga. This is a pointed allusion to the charioteer, his horses, and the chariot. One of the most famous parables in the Upanishads recalls and plays upon this root meaning:

> Know thou the soul (atman, self) as riding in a chariot,
> The body as the chariot.
> Know thou the intellect (buddhi) as the chariot-driver,
> And the mind (manas) as the reins.
>
> The senses (indriya), they say, are the horses;
> The objects of sense, what they range over. . . .
>
> He who has not understanding,
> Whose mind is not constantly held firm—

His senses are uncontrolled,
Like the vicious horses of a chariot-driver.

He, however, who has the understanding of a chariot-driver,
A man who reins in his mind—
He reaches the end of his journey,
The highest place of Vishnu.[1]

Yoking is accomplished in a wide variety of ways, depending on which school of yoga you follow. In *The Shambhala Encyclopedia of Yoga,* the scholar Georg Feuerstein catalogues nearly forty different schools of yoga suitable for different personalities or temperaments. Six schools are generally considered principal: classical or raja (royal), hatha (forceful), mantra (hymn), jnana (wisdom), bhakti (devotion), and karma (selfless action). It seems fitting that a word so closely associated with the meaning of union can embrace so many disparate schools.

While this union of the embodied self and the Great Self (paramaatman or brahman) is usually the stated goal of yoga practice, it's not always the case. The most prominent exception is the classical school of Patanjali, known as Raja-Yoga. Patanjali doesn't recognize a Great Self, though he does acknowledge a deity called the Lord (Ishvara), considered a special self (purusha-vishesha) among an infinite number regular selves (purusha). Patanjali defines classical yoga as the "restriction of the fluctuations of consciousness (Yoga-Sutra 1.2),"[2] which suggests the strenuous and risky job of harnessing itself, of bringing the skittish thoughts and rearing emotions under control.

However the supreme attainment is imagined, whether as a blissful merging with the Great Self or the quelling of the vicious horses of consciousness and nature, yogis emphasize both practice and study, especially study of sacred texts and self-study (svadhyaya, literally "going into one's own self"). Practice has two poles—an active pole that entails intense and persistent exertion (abhyasa) and a passive one that encourages what yoga tradition calls samatva, an attitude of evenness or equanimity toward the world. Yoga practice is a balancing act between doing and not-doing: we must somehow exhibit all the prowess of the charioteer in mastering his horses and yet remain the same whether in success or failure.

Yoga Practice

Many people tend to equate yoga merely with asana and know nothing about its underlying principles. But each school of yoga is founded on an integral vision of the world and the way it works, traced back to a divine source and so traditionally considered sacred and kept a closely guarded secret.

Each school's practice, then, its spiritual exertion or training, is a direct outgrowth of the original vision. The training and the vision together constitute a logical system. It's impossible to complete, or even understand the reason for, the training without first studying and contemplating the vision. Though outlined in guidebooks, the day-to-day training itself is conducted by an authority who has to some degree already realized the training's goal. Access to the training is limited to aspirants who are properly initiated into the school by the teacher after a period of apprenticeship. It's hard to remember sometimes how fortunate we are today to have easy access to any number of yoga guides in English translation.

Because it values the past, each school's system is inherently conservative or preservative. Training proceeds sequentially, in general stages (usually four), and each stage has its own special set of practices, which are considered congruous with the developmental level of the aspirant. The pace of the training is usually slow and steady. This slow pace ensures that the aspirant is ripe enough to receive each new practice. It's mostly futile and sometimes dangerous, the yogis believe, to proceed too quickly. Finally, the training is goal-oriented, and the goal is always liberation, whether conceived as yoking or harnessing, known as emancipation (apavarga, literally "to turn away") or aloneness (kaivalya).

A system like this has several advantages. It gives the aspirant a context, viewpoint (darshana), or map that shapes the way she looks at herself and the world, and a way for her to make sense of and express her experiences and insights. It also gets the aspirant up and moving, surrounds her with sympathetic fellow travelers, points her along well-marked paths, and outfits her with tried and true practical techniques agreeable to her personality and capacities.

But a system also has at least one serious drawback. Since it's a map, and not the territory itself, it's ultimately a limited way of seeing the world. While any one system approximates the truth, it's not the whole truth, just one way of perceiving it. A system can be an obstacle to growth and liberation, rather than a support, by dominating our perceptions and cramping our ability to accept or adapt to new information and experiences.

While formal training is the most common way we learn about yoga—and most students, at least at the beginning of their training, need the guidance and support of a system—it's definitely not the only way. Yoga also has an often unrecognized element of play, a word that's not typically associated with the practice. We like to think of ourselves as serious students and regard play as something childish, just playing the fool. But James Carse, in his book *Finite and Infinite Games,* reminds us that to be playful is not to be "trivial or frivolous, or to act as though nothing of consequence will happen. On the contrary, when we are playful with each other we relate as free persons, and the relationship is open to surprise; everything that happens is of consequence, for seriousness is a dread of the unpredictable outcome of open possibility. To be serious is to press for a specified conclusion. To be playful is to allow for possibility whatever the cost to oneself."[3]

According to some yogis, the world is the creation of the eternal feminine principle, the Goddess Shakti (power). The Sanskrit word for play, *lila,* also means "sport, diversion, amusement, pastime." This sacred play is a revelation of the very self-existence (svabhava) of the Goddess.

As opposed to training, true play is revolutionary. While tradition conserves and preserves, play turns over a new leaf, turns things upside down, stands things on their heads. We're urged to play around and not follow the rules, to take risks, to be spontaneous (child's play), open-ended (free play), experimental (play by ear), inventive. Play is accessible to everyone. If we recognize and revere the world as the play of the Goddess, we can join in and imitate this play in everything we do. Rather than distance ourselves from the world, in play we engage ourselves in the world and integrate it into the game. Play recognizes the inherent freedom and unique wisdom of the inner self. There's no outer authority, and so natural inclinations and the prompting of the inner self, not technique, impel our exertions. Finally, play is process-oriented and present-oriented. There's no future goal except to keep the play going.

While this guide will mostly stick to formal training, we'll kick up our heels every now and again and, instead of playing it safe, just play around. Keep your eyes open for these "Playing Around" sections sprinkled here and there in the chapters that follow. They will give you some ideas about how you, too, can play along with the Goddess.

Prana and Pranayama

If you pull pranayama apart, you'll find two smaller words, *prana* and *ayama*. *Prana* literally means "to breathe forth." It comes from the prefix *pra*, "to bring forth," and the verb *an*, "to breathe" or simply "to live." The entry for *prana* in my Sanskrit-English dictionary reads, "breath of life, breath, respiration, vitality, vigor, energy, power, and spirit."

Prana is a subtle energy that pervades every corner of the universe. While we can't see and touch it directly, at least not as beginning breathers, we can do so indirectly, through one of its most obvious physical manifestations and significant vehicles, our breath. As Lama Govinda writes in *Foundations of Tibetan Mysticism*, "As long as there is breath, there is life. We can do without all conscious functions of the mind and the senses for a comparatively long time, but not without breath. Breath therefore is the symbol of all the forces of life and stands first among the bodily functions of prana."[4]

The old guides agree that, just as each of us breathes along and so lives in and through prana, so, too, does the entire universe. "Like the spokes on the hub of a wheel," says a famous verse from the Prashna-Upanishad, "Everything is established on prana." This undifferentiated cosmic prana is called first prana (mukhya-prana) or whole prana (samasti-prana) (we'll look at what's called individual prana [vasti-prana] and its five branches in chapter 2).

In some old guides cosmic prana is one among several emanations or breathings of the Great Self. Suffused with its intelligence and creativity, prana isn't only the mainspring of all the various worlds, both physical and subtle, but their source and so master as well. "As a spider might come out with his thread, as small sparks come forth from the fire, even so from this Soul come forth all vital energies (prana), all worlds, all gods, all beings."[5] In other guides prana seems to be equated with the Great Self and by extension the embodied self itself: "The breathing spirit (prana) is Brahma . . . the intelligential self (prajnatman); [it is] bliss, ageless, immortal."[6] We can say, then, that prana creates, sustains, and illuminates the universe and links us to the source and essence of our lives. While we'll be working mostly with prana in its manifestation as the physical breath in this guide, always keep in mind that, unavoidably, we're also working with its subtle powers as well.

Ayama literally means "to stretch, extend; restrain, stop; expand, lengthen either in space or time." Interestingly its root word, *yama*, means "rein, curb, bridle; a driver, charioteer." Usually ayama is translated as "control," a word that has several denotations in English: to dominate, direct, regulate, and limit, in the sense of restrain. I caution you right away that you can't dominate the breath or the prana. As one of my students once said, trying to impose severe discipline on the breath invariably makes pranayama all the more difficult. But you can say that pranayama is the process of expanding our usually small reservoir of prana by lengthening, directing, and regulating the movement of the breath and then limiting or restraining the increased pranic energy in the body-mind.

The origin of pranayama, like the origin of just about all time-honored yoga practices, is obscure. Some scholars trace its lineage back to the Brahman priests who might have ministered to our charioteer's soul. These holy men had in their possession an extraordinary collection of hymns, prayers, incantations, and litanies, together called the Vedas. Veda means "knowledge." Its root word, vid, means "to know, understand, perceive, learn, have a correct notion of." This isn't the kind of knowledge we carry around in our heads, accumulated over the years, to help us manage the business of everyday life. Rather, it's knowledge revealed by the Great Self and heard (shruti) and then passed along by high-minded sages, knowledge that's considered eternal and infallible.

What's most remarkable to me about the Vedas is that, before the work assumed its written form some four thousand years ago, it was preserved entirely in the memories of the priests and transmitted orally from generation to generation. I have a translation of the oldest of the four main Vedic texts, the Rig-Veda, which runs to more than 650 pages with more than a thousand hymns. The priests were able to recite every syllable of this enormous hymnal without recourse to a written text. I think about this accomplishment every time I forget where I left my glasses or what I was supposed to buy at the grocery store.

As befitting their divine source, the hymns were always recited or sung with the utmost solemnity and concentration. Scholars speculate that, in order to say the words with the proper force and intonation, and so please the petitioned gods, the priests learned to regulate their breathing. In doing this, they discovered that when they changed their normal breathing rhythm to accommodate the rhythms of the hymns, they also changed their state of consciousness. This ritual regulation of the breath, scholars conclude, was the first step in the development of pranayama.

LAST WORD

However it got started, pranayama is a very refined practice today—after all, the yogis have had several thousand years to work it out and get it right. (We'll look more closely at two main schools of pranayama in chapter 2.) For now, remember that pranayama is a means of:

- Self-inquiry, since by looking at how we breathe, we begin to understand something about who we are.

- Self-transformation, since as the yogis say, breath and consciousness are really two sides of same coin, when we change the breath in pranayama, we inevitably change who we are.

- Self-realization, when our small breath becomes one with, and reveals itself as identical to, the Great Breath.

CHAPTER 2

Shining Forth

Truly, it is Life (prana) that shines forth in all things!
Understanding this, one becomes a knower.

—Mundaka-Upanishad,
The Thirteen Principal Upanishads

Breathing

Let's start our exploration of the yoga of breathing by asking an easy
question: Why do we breathe? We don't tend to think much about our
breathing. Why should we? Although we can influence the way we
breathe, breathing is largely an automatic process. Why be concerned
about something that seems to take care of itself just fine, when there
are so many other more important things to worry over?

But the answer to this question is fairly obvious. Breath, as we all
know, is life, an equivalence that's been recognized all over the
world for thousands of years. For example, remember that the word
prana is rooted in the verb *an*, which means "to breathe," but also
"to live" and "to move." In Sanskrit a *pranaka* is a living being. When
we stop breathing, at least for more than a few minutes, we stop
living. I'm sure you'll agree that this alone is a good enough reason
to keep on breathing. We breathe to take in and replenish the body's
store of oxygen for the production of energy in the body; maintain
balanced levels of oxygen and its essential partner, carbon dioxide,
in the body; and expel waste gases to purify the body.

So the why of breathing isn't much of a mystery, but let me ask you
another question you might not have considered before: How do
you breathe? Again, the answer seems obvious—with lungs and

diaphragm and nose and a few other things that we may not be quite sure about but that we're confident are working away to keep us alive. Obvious again.

But that's not exactly the answer I'm looking for. Maybe I should rephrase the question: How well do you breathe? You might believe that we all breathe in pretty much the same way and that it doesn't take a breathing genius to breathe well. But in fact, each of us has a unique breathing behavior or breathing identity. Some of us are very efficient breathers, while others—many others—aren't. Although it may not seem that important to be an efficient breather, inefficient breathing can have far-reaching consequences. Breathing experts cite three conditions in particular that contribute to inefficient breathing:

1. Poor posture, which might include a sagging spine and a stiff or sunken rib case.

2. Weak, uncoordinated, or constricted respiratory muscles, especially the diaphragm, our primary breathing muscle, and its breathing synergist, the rectus abdominis.

3. The wear and tear of everyday stress.

How does an inefficient breather breathe? She's inclined to breathe too shallowly, mostly high in the chest because the diaphragm is stuck, and too fast—she hyperventilates, which makes the flow of the breath turbulent. She often breathes through the mouth, which is universally censured because it reinforces hyperventilation, and under extreme stress she'll tend to hold her breath. Shallow, fast breathing reduces the carbon dioxide in the body, which constricts blood vessels and slows the circulation of blood and oxygen to the body and brain. Oxygen starvation chronically excites the sympathetic branch of the autonomic nervous system and the fight-or-flight response. So the heart beats rapidly or irregularly, she's by turns forgetful or confused, anxious or fearful, tense or irritable, and she's always tired and emotionally drained or flat.

On the other side of the ledger is the efficient breather. She breathes slowly, which streamlines the breath, with the free and easy movement of the diaphragm, engaging the entire torso (in fact, the entire body). She mostly breathes through the nose, which filters, warms or cools as needed, and humidifies the breath. Nose breathing naturally slows the exhale, because the nostrils offer more resistance to the breath than the mouth, and gives the lungs enough time to extract the maximum amount of oxygen and energy from each breath. With the correct proportion of oxygen and carbon dioxide in the body, which dilate the blood vessels, blood and oxygen circulate smoothly and easily through the efficient breather's body and brain. The full excursion of the diaphragm and the well-toned abdominals massage internal organs, like the heart and intestines, and so improve digestion and elimination. Efficient breathing activates the parasympathetic branch of the autonomic nervous system and the relaxation response. In all, the efficient breather is much calmer and more clearheaded, and probably healthier and happier, than her inefficient friend.

So how would you identify yourself as a breather? Efficient or inefficient, or somewhere in between? It's hard to answer a question like this objectively, especially when you might be a little fuzzy on the details of the function and machinery of breathing, with a breathing identity that's largely unexamined.

It's not surprising that the yogis have their own ideas about breathing. Of course, they're interested in efficient everyday breathing, but they're also interested in something more: not only why we breathe and how we breathe, but who is breathing.

We understand intuitively that breathing reflects consciousness and that we can affect or influence consciousness by changing our breath. We probably do it all the time and don't think much about it. For example, what happens to your breath when you get angry? Speeds up, right? And have you ever tried to soothe that anger by slowing down your breath? Probably, though it's not a sure thing. Just because you breathe slowly doesn't necessarily mean you're going to calm down, though it's a good start.

The point is, most of us don't think about the relationship between breath and consciousness and what it means. But luckily for us, the yogis do: it's their job. Thousands of years ago, they set about methodically investigating this relationship. They discovered that breath and consciousness are just the flip sides of the same coin and that in order to find out who is breathing, the first thing we need to do is ask how we breathe.

Individual Prana

Once the cosmic prana is appropriated into our body, it's converted into individual prana (vasti-prana), which has five major branches, usually called winds (vayu), collectively known as the great winds (maha-vayu). (There are also five minor branches, the upa-vayu, which won't concern us.) Each wind has its own special seat in the body (except circulating wind) and works to sustain us physically, mentally, and spiritually. Different teachers locate the seats of the winds in different areas of the body and give them different functions. For the purposes of this guide, we'll say that

- Forward wind (prana-vayu, not to be confused with cosmic prana) is seated in the heart and stimulates and regulates the rising energy of reaching out and taking in—that is, appropriation or absorption. Its primary manifestation, though not its only one, is inhalation.
- Downward wind (apana-vayu) is seated in the lower pelvis and stimulates and regulates the falling energy of elimination or giving out or away. Its primary manifestation (though, again, not its only one) is exhalation.
- Middle wind (samana-vayu) is the fire in the belly, seated in the navel, which stimulates and regulates assimilation or incorporation. Middle wind digests the food we take in from the world (with prana-vayu, whether physical, mental, or spiritual) and cooks it, as the yogis like to say, transmuting it into something uniquely our own.
- Circulating wind (vyana-vayu) circulates throughout our body and so has no specific seat. It's the glue that holds us together and the network that distributes what's been digested to every cell. Circulating wind also urges us to openly share what we've assimilated to ourselves with the body of the world.
- Upward wind (udana-vayu) is the energy of expression, appropriately seated in the throat. Lama Govinda (quoting René Guénon) notes that upward wind is a "vehicle of the mind, namely of word and speech, and thus, in a certain sense, the medium of an enlarged individuality."[1]

It's worth remembering that the five winds are not abstractions and not the preserve of just a few isolated yogis. They vitalize each of us, always and everywhere, whether we know it or not, with intelligence and creativity. Certainly, as beginning breathers, we can't be expected to immediately distinguish among these subtle currents and put them into play in our practice and lives. But wherever you are and whatever you're doing, it takes no particular training to begin to feel the great currents of aliveness that animate our body-mind. You just need to turn your attention, for a couple of minutes, to the movement of your everyday breathing.

Two Traditional Pranayama Models

Pranayama is referred to, mostly in passing without detailed instructions, in many of the old yoga guides. For example, in the Bhagavad-Gita, pranayama is mentioned as the balancing of the inhales and exhales (a technique we'll look at in chapter 17). "[All] contact with things outside he puts away, fixing his gaze between the eyebrows; inward and outward breaths he makes the same as they pass up and down the nostrils."[2]

Two models of pranayama have evolved over the centuries. The earlier one is the fourth limb of eight-limb yoga (ashta-anga-yoga), the central praxis of classical yoga or royal yoga (Raja-Yoga), outlined in the Yoga-Sutra, a well-known guide compiled by Patanjali sometime between eighteen hundred and twenty-two hundred years ago (modern scholars differ on its exact date). The later model belongs to Hatha-Yoga, which first appeared around 900 C.E., though like all yoga schools, its roots, such as Hindu Tantra and Indian alchemy, reach back centuries earlier. Its classical guidebook, written by Svatmarama Yogindra around the middle of the fourteenth century C.E., is the *Light on Forceful Yoga* (Hatha-Yoga-Pradipika). I'll also quote from two other Hatha-Yoga guides, *Gheranda's Collection* (Gheranda-Samhita) and *Shiva's Collection* (Shiva-Samhita), both products of the late seventeenth century C.E.

As I've mentioned, while many of us in the West equate yoga with asana, and while asana is certainly an important segment of classical and Hatha-Yoga, for the most part it's a preparation for pranayama and never practiced by itself. Svatmarama, for example, dedicates more than twice as many verses to pranayama as to posture. Posture practiced alone, without pranayama and meditation, surely has some physical value, but alone, it's not likely that it could ever lead to liberation.

Patanjali, Classical Yoga, and Pranayama

Classical yoga is credited with being the first systematic presentation of yoga, though most of the postures and breathing exercises with which we are familiar are products of Hatha-Yoga. Along with pranayama, the eight limbs include social and ethical obligations (yamas and niyamas), posture (asana), sensory inhibition (pratyahara), concentration (dharana), meditation (dhyana), and a remarkable state of identification or coalescence between the meditator and her object of meditation called samadhi (literally "putting together").

In Patanjali's guide there are 195 sutras (or 196 in some editions). Over the centuries many excellent commentaries have been written to supplement the sparse sutra style. The oldest surviving discussion (bhashya), written perhaps three hundred years after the Yoga-Sutra, is attributed to Vyasa, whose name means Compiler or Arranger. Vyasa is also recognized as the author of the four Vedas, the encyclopedic "tales of long ago" known as the Puranas, and the great Indian epic poem (at more than one hundred thousand verses, the longest in the world) the Mahabharata, which includes the Bhagavad-Gita. Since these texts evolved over more than three thousand years, either Vyasa was very old when he wrote his discussion or, more likely, there were a number of different sages over several generations named Vyasa.

We don't know much about Patanjali's life, although there's an interesting legend about his birth that relates that he fell (pat) from heaven into the open hands (anjali) of his virgin mother, Gonika. His yoga is essentially a rigorous program of behavior modification, attention training, and introverted self-inquiry, in which the practitioner invests all her energies in harnessing the turmoil, what Patanjali calls the fluctuations (vritti), of everyday consciousness (citta). You don't need to spend years meditating in a cave to get in touch with these fluctuations. Simply sit back, close your eyes for a few minutes, and train your awareness on your consciousness-stream. Then, to get a sense of the difficulty of harnessing this interior hurly-burly, try to focus on one thought or one object—even something as common as a pencil—for one minute, without straying from that focus at all. Unless you've been practicing meditation behind my back for a good while, I'll wager your best effort went awry after only a few seconds.

You might be thinking, So what's the problem? Who cares if I can't concentrate on a pencil for a minute? The problem, Patanjali says, is that we're identified with these fluctuations, that we believe they define—and so limit in time, space, will, knowledge, and capacity—who we are. But, he continues, these fluctuations are merely our surface self or camouflage, as the sage Sri Aurobindo calls it. "There is a personality on his [that is, the student's] surface that chooses and wills, submits and struggles, tries to make good in Nature or prevail over Nature, but this personality itself is a construction of Nature and so dominated, driven, determined by her that it cannot be free. It is a formation or expression of the Self in her, —it is a self of Nature rather than a self of Self . . . a temporary and constructed personality, not the true immortal Person."[3]

This identification—or more precisely, misidentification—with the surface self is called *avidya*. We've already run across a word related to avidya in chapter 1, veda, which you recall means "knowledge." Avidya literally means "not-knowing" or "not-seeing," and it's usually translated as "ignorance." It alienates us from our authentic self (purusha), which is "eternal, pure, joyful" (Yoga-Sutra 2.5), and so afflicts our lives with unrelenting suffering. Avidya, writes Heinrich Zimmer, "is the common doom of all living beings."[4]

The word Patanjali uses for suffering is *duhkha*, which literally means "having a bad axle hole." Doubtless in the days of chariots with wooden wheels and no shock absorbers, a bad axle hole could create a lot of suffering for a charioteer and his passenger. Patanjali suggests that each of us is like a misaligned wheel with a bad axle hole at the very core of our being, and it makes for an awfully bumpy ride.

The goal of classical yoga, then, can be simply stated: to "overcome the sorrow yet-to-come" (Yoga-Sutra 2.17) by stemming the tide of our fluctuations and resolving our unfortunate condition of ignorance. The method, as I've noted, is two-pronged: we must harness or restrict (nirodha) ever subtler levels of vrittis through committed practice or exertion (abhyasa) "cultivated properly and for a long time uninterruptedly" (Yoga-Sutra 1.14), while at the same time we must carefully discriminate (viveka) between what isn't and what is our authentic self and renounce (vairagya) the former and identify anew with the latter. All of this isn't as easy as it may seem. Like the charioteer's horses, the fluctuations aren't going to take our efforts to rein them in lying down. They seem to have a life of their own, and like all living things, they struggle to survive and express themselves.

Classical practice doesn't begin immediately with work on the citta-vrittis. Patanjali recognizes that's far too difficult. Instead, he instructs us to first grapple with fluctuations or movements that are more palpable and somewhat easier to harness, the movements of our body (in asana), breath (in pranayama), and senses (in pratyahara). You can see from its position in the hierarchy of limbs that pranayama can only begin after you've achieved some competency with asana, or posture, which is also true of pranayama in the Hatha model, and then is itself a preparation for sense inhibition and the three higher limbs of concentration, meditation, and samadhi.

Patanjali dedicates five sutras in the second chapter of his guide to pranayama. You can get a sense of the telegraphic sutra style by reading these lines without the bracketed words, all inserted by the translator (Yoga-Sutra 2.49–53):

> When this is [achieved, i.e. the mastery of posture], breath-control [which is] the cutting-off of the flow of inhalation and exhalation [should be practised]. [Breath-control is] external, internal and fixed in its movement, [and it is] regulated by place, time and number; [it can be] protracted or contracted. [The movement of breath] transcending the external and internal sphere is the fourth. Thence the covering of the inner light disappears. And [the yogin gains] the fitness of mind for concentration.

Classical pranayama is defined generally as the "cutting-off of the flow of inhalation and exhalation" (Yoga-Sutra 2.49); in other words, the classical aspirant strives to stop, or at least initially to greatly reduce, the movement of her breath. Remember that movement—any movement, including the movement of the body while breathing—is considered to be a fluctuation and so a distraction to meditation.

Patanjali recognizes three basic movements (vritti) or phases in each breathing cycle (Yoga-Sutra 2.50): external (bahya), or exhalation; internal (abhyantara), or inhalation; and fixed, or stopped (stambha). These are, of course, the same three movements of everyday breathing, though to be precise, there are really two stops or rests, one after the inhale and one after the exhale, and so four movements or phases. These three movements are in turn regulated by "place, time and number" (Yoga-Sutra 2.50):

- Place (desha) refers to the location in the body where the breath or prana is directed, such as the heart or the throat, though any place from the sole of the foot, says Vyasa, to the top of the head is suitable.

- Time (kala) is the duration of the inhalations and exhalations. Traditionally time is measured by repeating or reciting (japa) a sacred syllable or mantra (usually om) or by touching the tip of your thumb, in a particular pattern, to the twelve sections of the four digits, three on each finger, of the same hand. We'll break with tradition and use a modern convenience, a stopwatch.

- Number (samkhya) is the number of repetitions of the breathing cycles.

Patanjali mentions a fourth (caturtha) pranayama that transcends the three movements. The fourth is a state of arrested breathing that B. K. S. Iyengar calls kevala-kumbhaka, which means isolated or absolute retention. He characterizes it as "natural and non-deliberate," transcending the "sphere of breath which is modulated by mental volition,"[5] as opposed to the everyday breathing and the lower stages of pranayama, which all require varying degrees of effort and deliberation. (We'll look more closely at kumbhaka, or retention, in chapter 20.)

There's nothing in the Yoga-Sutra about the physical merits of pranayama. But Patanjali does record that it removes the covering of the inner light so that, as Bernard Bouanchaud comments, a "great lucidity, an unaccustomed sense of observation, and a quality of presence are very evident in one whose mental function has become transparent."[6] Classical pranayama, then, is primarily a technique for purifying consciousness and harnessing the citta-vrittis as a prelude to meditation.

Svatmarama, Hatha-Yoga, and Pranayama

Svatmarama's description of pranayama is considerably more detailed than Patanjali's. Patanjali only sketches the practice and its benefits in five sutras and expects a guru to provide the nuts and bolts of the teaching. Svatmarama, on the other hand, devotes much of his guide's second chapter and parts of the fourth to pranayama, though a guru is still needed to complete the practice. In the third chapter of the Pradipika, he also describes ten seals (mudra) and locks (bandha), which in general are specific muscular contractions of the body, hands, tongue, or mouth that serve to restrain, channel, and compress pranic energy and without which pranayama can't safely and successfully be practiced.

We usually think of Hatha-Yoga and classical yoga as being two very different traditions. But this distinction is only about four hundred years old. According to tradition, training in Hatha-Yoga is the first rung on the ladder leading to training in royal yoga.

But despite the old connection, there are significant differences between the theoretical viewpoints of classical yoga and Hatha-Yoga, and so in the kind of practices each favors and in the way the same practices are applied, including pranayama. (If this subject interests you, refer to "Recommended Readings," at the end of this guide.)

In classical yoga, nature (prakriti) and self (purusha) are eternally separate principles. Their strange relationship or correlation (samyoga), as Patanjali calls it, results in everyday consciousness (citta). Nature is essentially unintelligent, a clockwork process that exists only for the enjoyment and emancipation of the self. The self is pure consciousness that, unlike everyday consciousness (citta), has no content, no thoughts, emotions, memories, and desires. It simply watches, impassively, illuminating but not in any way participating in the myriad doings of prakriti. The classical deity, named the Lord (Ishvara), as a special purusha, also plays no active role in the everyday world. Classical practices are designed to free the self by divorcing it from its deluded association with nature. Once the self is liberated, nature—along with the yogi's body—no longer has a purpose, and so, as Patanjali states in his typically brisk way, is terminated.

In Hatha-Yoga pure consciousness is represented by a masculine God, Shiva (which means "benevolent" in Sanskrit). Like Patanjali's purusha and Ishvara, Shiva illuminates and witnesses, but never engages in, the grand and glorious play (lila) of feminine nature, the creation of and vehicle for the Goddess Shakti. But while purusha and prakriti are forever separate, correlated but never truly in contact, and while feminine prakriti exists only to serve masculine purusha (literally "man"), Shakti and Shiva are soul mates, separated in everyday thought only, but never in fact. Each of us is imbued with and sustained by the intelligence and creativity and bliss of both God and Goddess, and so each of us is a mirror for the world, both physical and subtle, reflecting in ourselves the eternal scheme of all Being and all Becoming.

Patanjali takes at best an arm's-length attitude toward the physical body. Hatha-Yoga seeks to nourish and preserve the physical vehicle and transform it into a divine body (divya-deha) or diamond body (vajra-deha), "lustrous and brilliant with a divine smell and diseaseless,"[7] with miraculous powers (siddhi) of its own.

The yogis often refer to our body, and more specifically the torso, as a pot (kumbha), which suggests the key role the body plays in the yoga of breathing as a container of vital energy, especially during the demanding practice of breath retention (kumbhaka, "potlike," which we'll look at in chapter 20). But the image also points to the need to ready the body for pranayama. The untrained body is like an unbaked clay pot. Just as such a pot would dissolve if filled with water, so would such a body break down if suddenly charged with an unaccustomed jolt of vital energy. The body, just like the pot, must be fired and tempered before it's a fit receptacle. "No sickness, no old age, no death has he / Who has obtained a body made out of the fire of Yoga."[8]

The body is crisscrossed from head to toe with nadis. "The term Nadi comes from the root 'Nad' which means motion. . . . If they were revealed to the eye the body would present the appearance of a highly complicated chart of ocean currents. Superficially the water seems one and the same. But examination shows that it is moving with varying degrees of force in all directions."[9] Nadi is translated in various ways, such as "channel, conduit, vessel, vein, artery, nerve." The word refers both to actual nerves, veins, and arteries in the physical body, which are known to medical science, and to subtle energy channels, sometimes called yoga-nadis, in the subtle body through which the vayus circulate.

The number of channels in the body is a matter of debate. According to different guides, there may be 350,000 or 300,000 or 72,000 or 101. These numbers should not be taken too literally. They simply indicate that there are countless channels. The entire network is sometimes called the wheel of channels (nadi-cakra).

The origin of the channels is also disputed. In some guides they originate in the heart and spread out, like the tendrils of a vine, in all directions.

> There are a hundred and one channels of the heart.
> One of these passes up to the crown of the head.
> Going up by it, one goes to immortality.
> The others are for departing in various directions.[10]

Other guides assert that the channels originate in an egg-shaped bulb (kanda) located sometimes near the base of the spine, sometimes in the middle of the body. The Hatha-Yoga-Pradipika, for example, locates the bulb just above the anus and says that it appears to be covered with soft, white cloth.

However many channels the various guides recognize and wherever they originate, only fourteen are generally considered important, and of these three are chief. The central channel, called the most gracious channel (sushumna-nadi) or the middle (madhya), follows the center of the spinal column from an opening in the bulb, called the Brahma gate (brahma-dvara), to the Brahma fissure (brahma-randhra, the sutura frontalis) or Brahma cave (brahma-bila) at the crown of the head. Sushumna, you could say, is a channel from the small self to the Great Self through the core or middle of our being.

The other two channels also originate in the bulb and spiral upward around this central channel in a dance of life, distributing their force throughout the body in the service of material existence (see fig. 2.1). It's often remarked that these three together form what we in the West call a caduceus, the winged Hermes staff with the twined serpents. The channel spiraling upward from the base of the spine and ending at the left nostril is the comfort channel (ida-nadi), which represents the feminine and the dark side of consciousness and is appropriately symbolized by the moon. Its entwined mate, which ends at the right nostril, is the tawny or reddish channel

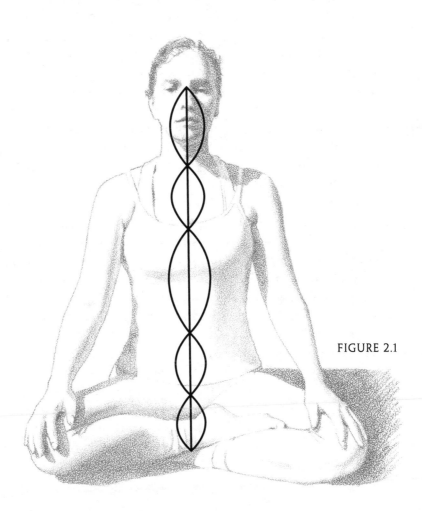

FIGURE 2.1

(pingala-nadi), which is the masculine and bright side of consciousness, symbolized by the sun. The three channels meet at six
places along the spine: the base of the spine, the lower abdomen,
navel, heart, throat, and center of the forehead. Each confluence
of the channels marks the site of an energy center, called a wheel
(cakra, sometimes spelled chakra, and pronounced with a hard ch,
as in church) or lotus (padma). The channels join for the last time
in the center of the forehead, where they form a knot called the
triple braid of release (mukta-triveni) or the triple peak (tri-kuta).
From here ida and pingala pass to the left and right nostrils, respectively, while the sushumna continues on to the crown.

As a beginning breather, don't worry too much about these subtle wheels and channels. For now just remember that the wheels are
both "certain locations of energies in the body," as Ken Wilber
writes, and "certain stages in a type of spiritual growth (steps in the
freeing up of transcendent bliss)."[11] The three lowest are commonly
thought of as self-centered—that is, concerned with self-preserva-
tion and self-survival, self-continuance in procreation, and self-pro-
jection of power into the world. The fourth wheel, at the heart, is
seen as a transition from totally self-centered concerns to concerns
about embracing the world. The fifth wheel represents worldly
knowledge and the beginning of self-knowledge; and the sixth
wheel, spiritual insight.

After Shakti fashions the world, she divides. Part of her remains
active as the life force, or prana, and part of her takes up residence
at the base of the spine, where she falls asleep, no doubt tuckered
out by the prodigious exertions of world building. In this state she's
usually pictured as a sleeping serpent, looped in $3\frac{1}{2}$ coils, and so
called the coiled one, or kundalini. Both asleep and coiled like a
spring, the serpent is a symbol of our own spiritual slumber (avidya)
and potential.

The goal of Hatha-Yoga is to unite (or reunite, rather than separate)
consciousness and nature. In the average person the prana-vayus diffuse throughout all the nadis save sushumna, the entrance to which
is said to be blocked by the mouth of the slumbering serpent (some
authorities hold that there's a trickle of prana in sushumna). Consciousness, then, is said to be externalized, involved solely in the outer
world and ignorant of its vast spiritual reservoir. In this ignorance,

in which the sun and moon, represented by pingala and ida, are active and sushumna is obstructed, these folks are subject to day and night, by which the yogis mean time, suffering, and physical death.

The yogis gather this vital energy and withdraw it from everyday life, then direct it toward the dormant spiritual life nascent at the root-foundation (muladhara). They next heat the concentrated prana and through this arouse the sleeping kundalini, which is said to climb, hissing, through the sushumna-nadi from the base of the spine, through progressively subtler levels of existence, to the thousand-spoked wheel (sahasrara-cakra) at the crown of the head. Here Shakti joins in a sacred marriage with Shiva, and the yogi enters samadhi, which is said to consume time and death and lead to self-realization, immortality, and liberation.

The Benefits of Pranayama

The old guides list a large number of benefits—physical, psychological, and spiritual—for pranayama. Of course, this list is based on the authors' practical experiences and the collected wisdom of their schools and can't be considered scientific evidence, at least by our modern Western standards. But some of the reported physical benefits seem tenable and not beyond the reach of most assiduous aspirants. For example, pranayama is said to stoke the gastric fire, which improves digestion and speeds elimination of wastes from the body, and appease thirst and hunger so you won't be distracted by these cravings during practice; open the sinuses to allow more air into the body; purify both the gross and subtle energy systems of the body; and cure many diseases and conditions, including nervous disorders, indigestion, cough, and fever.

But we might take some other benefits only with a grain or two of salt. For example, Svatmarama notes somewhat enthusiastically that pranayama will make you look as if you're a teenager again and improve your love life. I've been practicing now for nearly twenty years, and I'm afraid I can't lend any credence to this last assertion, though it does strongly encourage me to practice regularly. I'm also spurred on by claims—though again, the jury's still out on them— that pranayama promotes extraordinary mental and physical powers, such as clairvoyance and levitation; engenders indescribable happiness; awakens the sleeping serpent kundalini, which leads to living liberation (jivan-mukti); and best of all, destroys death. "Even Brahma and other gods in heaven devote themselves to practising pranayama because it ends the fear of death."[12]

Realistically, as a beginning breather, what benefits can you expect from pranayama? It's hard to generalize, of course, because as with anything else, what you get out of the practice depends on how much you put into it. To realize any benefits, it's crucial to commit to a regular practice and cultivate it properly. Also, some students take to the practice like fish to water. You could say, if you're in a yogic frame of mind, that these aspirants have good breathing karma. To other students, though, the practice is about as enjoyable as an appointment with the dentist or a letter from the IRS. So to be on the safe side, it's best to have relatively moderate expectations about your practice, at least for the first year or so. Transcendent bliss and eternal life, I would venture, are probably not in the cards. But based on my own experience and the experiences of my students, there are some benefits in particular that you can reasonably anticipate.

It's not unlikely, first of all, that you'll become more aware of, and gain greater control over, your everyday breath. Why is this a benefit? It's well known and widely accepted that your breath and your mental states are closely related, that the former reflects and can be used, to a certain extent, to influence the latter. I suppose we've all, at one time or another, taken a few deep breaths to calm an angry outburst or to suck up a little extra energy when feeling weary. Certainly yoga has recognized the importance of this connection of breath and consciousness (citta) for hundreds of years. Svatmarama, for example, writes that "when prana moves, chitta (the mental force) moves. When prana is without movement, chitta is without movement. By this (steadiness of prana) the yogi attains steadiness. . . ."[13] With the instrument of your breath, then, you can monitor and modulate your psychic temperature throughout the day, cooling yourself down when the mental mercury rises and heating yourself up when it drops. Many of my students have reported that pranayama made them more relaxed overall and increased their store of energy, not only for yoga practice in general but also for the business of their everyday lives. I have the sense, now that I've developed a pretty consistent awareness of my breath during the day, that I'm practicing pranayama pretty much all the time (at least when I'm awake) and that I can watch myself—and so get to know myself better—from moment to moment, no matter what I'm doing.

There's also a good chance that your everyday breathing will become slower; in other words, you'll take fewer breaths throughout the day. The benefit here? You'll expend less energy in the lifelong enterprise of breathing and so have more energy to direct toward other pursuits—such as asana practice. As your breathing slows, it will also smooth out, which is a kind of natural relaxant for the stresses and strains of our breathlessly paced world. All of this is to say that your breathing will become less effortful, more efficient.

LAST WORD

Of course, there are potential benefits for your yoga practice, too, a couple of which I've already suggested. I read somewhere once— I don't remember where, though I suspect it was in something that Mr. Iyengar wrote—that pranayama acts like a "jackhammer" on tight muscles, especially in the chest. I've found that pranayama, more like a crowbar than a jackhammer, has slowly pried open some (though, I must admit, not all) of the tighter places in my body and so provided me with new openings in my asana practice. This, in turn, affects my breathing, and so on and so on, asana and pranayama oscillating back and forth to each other's advantage.

CHAPTER 3

Obstacles and Helpers
Antaraya and Pari-karman

> The obstacles that distract thought are disease, apathy,
> doubt, carelessness, indolence, dissipation, false vision,
> failure to attain a firm basis in yoga, and restlessness.
>
> —Patanjali, *Yoga: Discipline of Freedom:*
> *The Yoga Sutra Attributed to Patanjali,*
> translated by Barbara Stoler Miller

Obstacles (Antaraya)

Three hundred years ago the anonymous author of the Shiva-Samhita cautioned his students that "there are many hard and almost insurmountable obstacles in Yoga, yet the Yogi should go on with his practice at all hazards; even were his life to come to the throat."[1] He was telling them that a trip into the county of the Self isn't always easy. Some days, just as on any other trip, there are obstacles to overcome: either it's raining outside, the locals aren't very friendly, or you take a wrong turn and get lost.

But while I agree with the author that you should always press on with your practice no matter what obstacle arises, I'm not sure that struggling until your life comes to your throat is wise. At the very least, you'd have a really hard time breathing. There's no denying that yoga practice can be frustrating or maddening at times, but a life-and-death struggle with obstacles usually just makes things worse.

In a sense, obstacles are defense mechanisms. They're a part of ourselves protecting us from ourselves and preventing us from pushing our practice along too quickly. These defense mechanisms becomes obstacles only when:

- We quit and walk away from yoga entirely.

- We ignore the obstacle, either consciously or unconsciously, and banish from our practice the cause (or causes) that seems to precipitate it.

- We confront the obstacle head-on, like a battering ram, with face and eyes and teeth set in a determined grimace, and struggle to get around or over or through it as quickly as possible.

Most of us are accustomed to doing something when we feel thwarted, to fix the problem or at least tinker with it to make it better. While it's appropriate at times to push against an obstruction, more often than not, this strategy leads to frustration or, worse, to injury.

The Sanskrit word for obstacle is *antaraya*, which means "to come between." Obstacles come in many shapes and sizes, both physical and mental. In classical yoga antarayas are vritti-factories that continually churn out impediments to practice. Fortunately for us, the yogis catalogued dozens of obstacles in their guides, mostly of the mental kind, that come between us and our destination. They've done this to alert us to possible detours and stumbling blocks on the road ahead, reassure us that obstacles are natural features of the practice landscape, and encourage us to press on and not get dispirited.

Probably the best-known traditional obstacles are the nine listed in the first chapter of the Yoga-Sutra (1.30). The first, sickness (vyadhi), is a physical obstacle, but the other eight can be considered mental. These include languor (styana), doubt (samshaya), heedlessness (pramada), sloth (alasya), dissipation (avirati), false vision (bhranti-darshana), nonattainment of yogic stages (alabdha-bhumikatva), and instability in these stages (anavasthitatva).

Patanjali adds that his obstacles are attended by four distractions (vikshepa): suffering or pain (duhkha), depression or melancholy (daurmanasya), physical restlessness (angam-ejatva), and disturbed breathing. These distractions are surefire signs that something is wrong with our practice, whether it's pranayama or posture, or almost anything else.

I don't believe that Patanjali had to contend with all nine obstacles in his own practice. At least I hope not. It seems more likely he collected them in conversations with colleagues and students, and from his school's tradition, both written and oral. Over the years I've collected accounts of dozens of obstacles, both physical and mental, from my students' journals.

Physical Obstacles

There are three general categories of physical obstacles. We'll work with the first two as we go through the guide: (1) ignorance about the topography of the body and the qualities of the breath; (2) imbalance and its related tension, found just about anywhere in the body; and (3) sickness, usually a cold or the flu and accompanying symptoms of misery and despair. Depending on the severity of this sickness, your pranayama practice should be modified to a simple reclining breathing awareness or put on hold altogether until you feel better.

Mental Obstacles

There are also eight mental obstacles that seem to surface again and again:

Dismay. Many beginning breathers feel dismayed by the prospect of mastering an entirely new practice from scratch. One student told me, after sitting in on a few classes and thumbing through *Light on Pranayama*, "There's just so much to learn." At the time I thought he was excited by the prospect of adding to his store of yoga knowledge. It turned out that he was simply put off by the wealth or welter of information and practices.

Indolence. Sometimes called sloth, inertia, or laziness, indolence is probably the most common obstacle. Almost all of us, however many years we've been trudging along in our practice, struggle occasionally (or more than occasionally) with indolence, our built-in resistance (tamas) to doing our daily work.

The urgent need to justify indolence, by the way, to ourselves and others, occasions some of the most creative journal entries I get.

Exotic vacations, visits from long-lost relatives, protracted bouts with strange diseases, child-rearing responsibilities, life-shattering career or residence changes, alien abductions—all seem to increase dramatically during the usual eight-week run of my pranayama course.

Distraction. Many students find they can't relax and focus on the breath because they're too distracted by the fluctuations of their consciousness.

Discouragement, impatience, doubt. Students often report that, even after they practice diligently for several months, absolutely nothing happens or that, at least in their opinion, things happen too slowly. This experience usually leads to one of three different obstacles:

The student gets discouraged. Compared to posture, pranayama seems to require an effort out of all proportion to the results.

The student gets impatient. Even Mr. Iyengar describes pranayama as tedious and repetitive. As one student complained, "All this lying around on blankets is a big waste of time." Someone like this will frequently skip over the foundation practices and plunge headfirst into "real" pranayama. In his haste he may well trip over an obstacle I call "incapacity," which is trying to do something you're not really prepared to do.

But most commonly the student starts to doubt. There are two kinds of doubt. In the first kind the student may doubt the practice of yoga itself, either because he has the wrong teacher or the wrong approach for his needs or temperament or because the practice seems ineffective in the face of a seemingly insurmountable obstacle, to borrow a phrase from the Shiva-Samhita.

The second kind of doubt is self-doubt. Here, when faced with that insurmountable obstacle, the student doubts not the efficacy of the practice but his own capacities. Faith in the practice can be restored, in the first instance, by finding a more simpatico teacher or practice environment, or maybe a different book. The other two varieties of doubt are more difficult to overcome. They seem to dampen the student's interest in the practice and his willingness to continue the journey.

The cautious lions, elephants, and tigers approach to pranayama is especially susceptible to these three obstacles. It's never easy to make an effort without having something to show for that effort. But the fact is that pranayama, for most students, develops much more slowly than posture. It's important to understand this at the outset of your journey and lower your expectations accordingly.

Instability. Not all beginners report difficulties early in their practice. "I've never done anything as incredible as this before," exclaimed one student. "It's changing my whole life." But it sometimes happens that after this promising start, the student slips back to what he considers to be a lower level of practice. Patanjali calls this instability or unsteadiness (anavasthitatva).

Instability isn't an obstacle if the student accepts the backward step as simply a phase in the natural ebb and flow of all spiritual adventure. But after tasting nothing but the sweetness of the practice at the outset, it's difficult to lose that flavor or have it turn bitter. She's then prone to quit the practice in frustration.

Fear. The last obstacle is, I think, the most formidable of all and so the most threatening to the continuation of our breathing practice. It can appear anytime, early on or later down the road, and usually with no warning. For convenience I call it fear, but in fact, students' reactions vary, and as a descriptive word, fear may be too strong for some or too weak for others.

We often forget that pranayama isn't merely deep breathing. Instead, it's a powerful means of penetrating avidya. Remember, Patanjali tells us that, through pranayama, the veil that covers the light of our higher awareness (buddhi) is lifted.

Sometimes the light illuminates things that are truly awesome and wondrous. Other times, though, the light is far too bright, and it shines into the darker corners of our consciousness, where we discover things about ourselves we'd rather not know. It's important to remember that inefficient breathing often reinforces the bridling of unpleasant or dangerous thoughts or emotions. When we change the way we breathe and make it more efficient, these thoughts or emotions frequently rise to the surface of our awareness.

Truthfully, while the fear seems threatening, it's really a signal that our practice is on track and working as advertised. It tells us that we're cutting through the coverings of avidya, the innate and acquired structures and agents of our consciousness, especially our surface self, that obscure our authentic self.

Sometimes, depending on the nature of the insight, the student can face the fear. If she's willing to accept that self-knowledge isn't always comfortable and keep going, her practice usually becomes stronger and more self-assured.

PRELIMINARY

What's the best way to deal with obstacles, then? Even before you begin your journey and start meeting obstacles, do three things. First, inquire honestly of yourself, Am I truly ready for pranayama? Think about what's involved in the practice before you commit to it. Recognize that pranayama is an everyday practice that demands time and effort and may not return any rewards for weeks or months to come. Many students realize that, after a few weeks of half-hearted practice, they don't really feel fit for (adhikara) the work. They may not be interested in breathing, they may not have the time for—or be willing to spend the time on—another responsibility in their lives, or they may not see the point of the practice. Whatever. The real obstacle to these students' practice is that they don't want to practice in the first place.

What do you do if you discover that you're not ready, especially after investing your hard-earned money in this guide? Don't worry. The best policy is simply to let the practice go for the time being and put this guide on the shelf. Don't sell it back to the bookstore at half price quite yet, though. Continue to work on your postures and always end your sessions with a long Corpse (shavasana; see chapter 8). Be patient. If you're sincere about yoga, someday you'll no doubt feel ripe to begin pranayama and pull this guide down off the shelf again.

But if you are ready to start, then the next step is to gracefully accept your ignorance. Allow that you don't know everything there is to know about yourself or that things you think you know about yourself may be mistaken. I have a mantra I repeat to myself now and again, just as a reminder of this: "I don't know who I am." By admitting ignorance immediately and willingly, you weaken its grip on your consciousness and are more accepting of whatever obstacles come along.

Some students resent being asked to concede they're ignorant. Don't forget, this ignorance has nothing to do with your IQ and doesn't necessarily make you a bad person. Even smart people and people who do good deeds are bound by avidya. Think of it as a kind of metaphysical blind spot intrinsic to everyone's everyday consciousness.

Finally, when you're ready to commit to practice and you've accepted your ignorance, ask yourself the most important question of all: Do I truly want to know who I am? This question logically follows from our ignorance, but it also issues from an intense desire that all of us have to know the truth about ourselves and what the yogis call a longing for liberation (mumukshutva). This is, as the sage Shankara wrote eleven hundred years ago, the "will to be free from the fetters forged by ignorance . . . through the realization of one's true nature."[2]

We don't always recognize how essential this desire is to our practice. It's common for beginning students to think that yoga is something they do, that it's apart from who they are. Their practice, then, is not integral to their being and is often haphazard and mechanical. More experienced students, though, usually recognize that their practice expresses who they are, that it flows out from their being to sustain and replenish their lives.

Just as prana is the hub of the wheel of life, the mantra "Who am I?" is truly the hub of all spiritual practice. As the great sage Ramana Maharshi said, "Every living being longs always to be happy, untainted by sorrow; and everyone has the greatest love for himself, which is solely due to the fact that happiness is his real nature. Hence, in order to realize that inherent and untainted happiness . . . it is essential that he should know himself. For obtaining such knowledge the enquiry Who am I? in quest of the Self is the best means."[3]

Some students discover that they don't really want to know. There's also a part of everyone's nature that's comfortable with the status quo and that doesn't like change. It might be useful, even at this early stage, to jot down a few impressions about your response to the big question, Who am I? Don't worry about being right or wrong; give yourself permission to speculate and have fun. Hold on to your jottings for later, when you start writing in your journal (see chapter 6), the report about your trip through the country of the Self. You can enter what you've written as a kind of prologue. It will remind you of where you started from and, as you wend your way over hill and dale, how far you've traveled.

But even students who are well prepared for the journey run into obstacles. After all, they're ignorant, too. And while well-prepared students do struggle occasionally and even quit their practice, I've noticed that they tend to treat their obstacles not as foes to yoga, as Vyasa says, but as opportunities to further their practice.

With the help of their Witness and the four projections (bhavanata) listed by Patanjali—friendliness (maitri), compassion (karuna), gladness (mudita), and equanimity (upeksha or samatva)—they first carefully look at the obstacle from every angle over a period of days, weeks, or months, depending on the obstacle. They don't do anything but simply observe and gather as much information as they can about the obstacle and their reaction to it. Frequently, when this choiceless awareness (a phrase coined by J. Krishnamurti) is applied to the problem, the obstacle itself seems to suggest an opportune solution.

Helpers (Pari-karman)

You might expect that the yogis wouldn't leave us hanging out there on the obstacle limb without any help, and you would be right. Patanjali, for one, comes to our rescue with a number of different helpers to whom we can turn for succor whenever the obstacles seem to be piling up to Himalayan heights. In addition to the four projections mentioned above, he mentions several other helping hands, such as:

- Faith in the rightness of what you're doing and in the certainty of your own success. Faith is bolstered by energy (virya) and enthusiasm in the original sense of the word, which is to be inspired or possessed (entheos) by a god. "The person who has control over himself attains verily success through faith; none other can succeed. Therefore, with faith, the Yoga should be practiced with care and perseverance."[4]

- Clear intention and constant mindfulness (smirti) of what you're doing and why, in regard to both short-term and long-term goals and in the subtle adjustments of everyday practice.

- Contentment (samtosha), which accommodates both success and failure with good humor and grace, and self-acceptance; at the same time, the willingness to take risks and embrace uncertainty. "As long as one is not satisfied in the self, he will be subjected to sorrow. With the rise of contentment the purity of one's heart blooms. The contented man who possesses nothing owns the world."[5]

- Careful discrimination (viveka) between what's important to your practice and what's not, and the willingness to surrender the latter.

- Open-minded study (svadhyaya) of traditional and contemporary guides to breathing and yoga, and associating with and contemplating on what Patanjali calls the vita-ragas, the beings who have conquered attachment. "By listening to instructions, by contemplation and by being in the company of a calm and sure-minded preceptor, doubts can be removed."[6]

Not only Patanjali but virtually every authority on pranayama emphasizes the need for regular, sustained, patient practice. "Perfect consciousness is gained through practice. Yoga is attained through practice; . . . through practice is gained success in pranayama."[7]

LAST WORD

Don't be surprised—or discouraged or doubtful—if you discover some antaraya that I haven't mentioned in this chapter. The ones I've listed here are just among the most common and surely don't exhaust all the possibilities—the flat tires, delayed flights, missed connections, and whatever else the universe and your karma cook up to make the journey interesting and exciting. Be assured that whatever obstacles you unearth, in the thousands of years that yoga has been practiced, other aspirants have bumped into them, too, and lived to tell the tale.

By the same token, I haven't listed all the pari-karman either. While the universe often seems as if it's out to get you, the yogis have an abiding faith in its goodness and grace as well as an abiding faith that its fondest wish is for you to be happy and know yourself. Keep your eyes and ears and heart vigilant for helpers. Just as the obstacles lead to the four distractions (vikshepa), the helpers take us to their opposites: the discharge of sorrow and pain, contentment, steadiness of the body-mind, and—best of all—easy breathing.

CHAPTER 4

Props

I first used a prop in 1948 when I was not getting Baddha Konasana at all. I started using bricks, the heavy stones which were available in the street.

—B. K. S. Iyengar replying to a question about props, from "A Visit with B. K. S. Iyengar," *Iyengar: His Life and Work*

MY DICTIONARY defines a prop as an object that's placed beneath or against a structure to keep it from falling or shaking. My daughter's first two-wheel bicycle came with a pair of little outrigger training wheels, which served two purposes: they allowed her to do something right away—stay upright on the bike—that she wasn't otherwise yet ready to do and gave her a feel for what balancing on two wheels would be like, down the road when the training wheels came off. When her skill and confidence increased to a critical level, we removed the training wheels, and after a few minor shakes, off she charged on two wheels without falling.

I suppose that we've all used props at one time or another, to keep ourselves or things around us from falling or shaking. Yogis use props, too, and though we may think of them as being a relatively recent innovation, they have actually been around for centuries. Gheranda, for example, describes how to wrap a yoga cloth (yoga-patta) around your outer legs and pelvis to help support a cross-legged posture during meditation or pranayama: "Encircling the loins with a piece of cloth, seated in a secret room. . . . One cubit long, and four fingers wide should be the encircling cloth, soft, white and of fine texture."[1]

Probably the foremost contemporary advocate of yoga props is

B. K. S. Iyengar, who's been developing a kind of science of props now for more than fifty years. Teachers trained in his approach learn to apply the basic principles of this science in lots of different situations, both in public classes for their everyday students, whether at beginning or intermediate levels, and in therapeutic work with injured or disabled students. Much like my daughter's training wheels, yoga props provide an immediate support in an exercise or a posture in the form of bracing, pressure, resistance, lengthening, release, or lift. This enlightens dark or unexplored areas of the body or intensifies our awareness of familiar areas. Props can be used in both active and passive situations. In a passive posture, the prop enables us to hold an approximate position a lot longer than we ordinarily might be able to. Props also give us an experience of future possibilities by allowing us to perform an exercise or a posture that would otherwise be difficult or impossible and so approach the approximate experience of the completed posture. This educates our brain and muscles about what's needed in the posture; expands the normally perceived, and often unnecessarily limited, boundaries of our body image and movement repertoire; and prepares for the day when we can stand on our own two feet.

I should mention that props do have critics. Props, they say, too easily become crutches that create dependency and so, instead of moving us along the path toward self-sufficiency and self-understanding, actually block the way. This point is well taken, and I think it's important to recognize and appreciate this potential prop pitfall. However, used judiciously and, as we progress in our practice, with less and less frequency, props are an enormous boon.

If you're not accustomed to using props, you might feel a bit awkward or uncomfortable with them at first. Give them a chance. Don't be reluctant to experiment with the props described here or even devise new ones of your own. After all, experimenting and improvising are exactly what Mr. Iyengar has been doing for a half century and what the yogis have done for many millennia.

In each of the following sections, you'll find a simple introductory description of a prop; what you can use to stand in for the prop in a pinch and how you can, if possible, make the prop yourself; and how you'll generally use the prop.

Blanket

Yoga blankets are made of wool or cotton, or a blend of one of these and synthetic materials. A yoga blanket is used primarily as a support, either for the spine and torso when reclining or for the buttocks when sitting. When fully open, they measure about 4½ to five feet by seven feet, but for our purposes, the blanket will be folded in various ways. For convenience of description, we'll use the following blanket terminology when folding: by matching the short edges, we'll fold widthwise; and by matching the long edges, we'll fold lengthwise.

Take your blanket now and fold it widthwise three times: you'll have a rectangle that measures about twenty inches by thirty inches. Look at the two short edges of the rectangle. One edge is sharp, where the blanket was folded over on itself on the second fold and then doubled on the third. The other edge is dull, where the sides of the blanket were matched during folding (see fig. 4.1).

If you're serious about your practice, you should have three to four blankets. However, in an emergency, alternatives include several thick bath towels or a firm pillow or cushion.

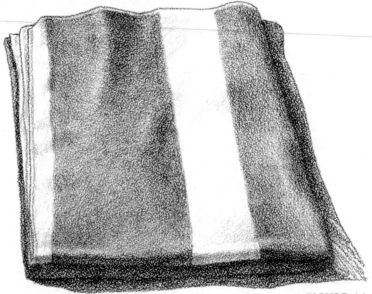

FIGURE 4.1

Bolster

Two different shapes of cotton-stuffed bolsters are available. The round bolster is about two feet in length by eight or nine inches in diameter (see fig. 4.2). The rectangular bolster is about thirty inches by fourteen inches by three inches thick. A bolster is useful, though not essential. Acceptable alternatives include a rolled-up blanket or bath towel or a firm pillow or cushion. Like a rolled or folded blanket, a bolster is used mostly for reclining support, either for a warm-up exercise or for breathing.

A pranayama bolster is distinct from a regular bolster. As its name suggests, it is a special support for pranayama, though it can be used for other purposes. It's a skinny version of the round bolster, about thirty inches long, eight inches wide, and four inches in diameter. Like the round bolster, a pranayama bolster is not essential. Acceptable alternatives include a rolled-up blanket or bath towel or a firm pillow or cushion. A pranayama bolster serves as a support for the spine and torso when you practice reclining pranayama.

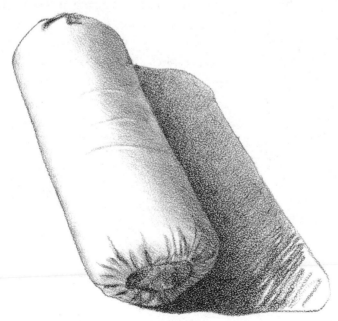

FIGURE 4.2

Block

Most yoga blocks are made of wood. But blocks are now also made of foam, which is much lighter and safer—if you happen to drop one on your foot or head—than wood. A block provides support, resistance, and tactile aid. A typical block measures nine inches by five inches by three inches. Have one or two on hand (see fig. 4.3).

For convenience of description, we'll use the following block terminology:

> The block has two ends, which measure three by five inches.
>
> Two sides, which measure three by nine inches.
>
> Two faces, which measure five by nine inches.
>
> The long axis of the block is its length (nine inches), while its short axis is its width (five inches).

Though I'm not enthusiastic about the idea, a book or bound stack of books is often suggested as a viable alternative to a block. You can also make your own block. Get a piece of wood measuring about five inches by three inches and saw off something like a nine-inch-long piece. Be sure to sand the wood, especially the sharp corners and edges, or cover the block with tape.

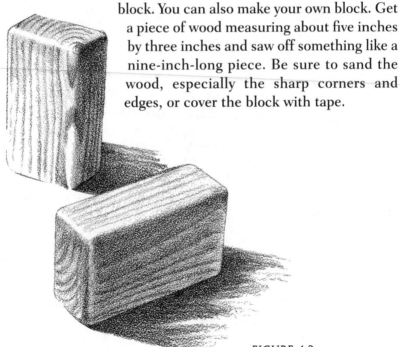

FIGURE 4.3

Strap with Buckle

Yoga straps are usually made of stiff cotton. Yogis like to tie themselves up in various ways with straps. I know this sounds strange, but trust me, it's perfectly OK. Yoga straps are about six feet long and one to three inches wide and have either a metal or a plastic buckle. Have one or two on hand (see fig. 4.4).

When you bind a body part, or bind two or more parts together, it's usually much easier to adjust a buckled strap. You have to knot an unbuckled strap around the part or parts, and it's often difficult to get just the right tightness. But acceptable alternatives include a necktie, usually two or three knotted together; a piece of sturdy cloth like denim or corduroy cut to the above measurements; or a gi belt, which can be bought at a martial arts school or supply store. You can also make your own buckled belt with a length of strap and a plastic buckle (the snap-release kind work well), both of which you can buy at a camping supply store.

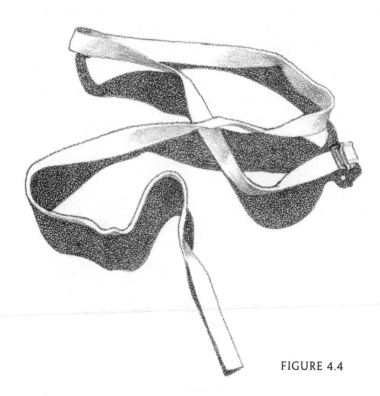

FIGURE 4.4

Sandbag

Yoga bags are usually called sandbags, though they're seldom filled with sand nowadays. The bag itself is commonly made of some sturdy material, like canvas, and is filled with very fine gravel. Sandbags are used to weigh things down. Bags from different makers have slightly different dimensions, but generally a bag measures about fourteen to eighteen inches by six to eight inches and weighs ten pounds. You'll need one or two (see fig. 4.5).

A possible alternative is a doughnut-shaped, iron barbell weight, which you can buy in a sporting goods store for a few dollars. These weights will work for many exercises but not for all, and compared to a bag, they can be uncomfortable—and very cold to the touch—and hard to manage. You can also make your own bag, if you have a sewing machine or know someone who does. Sew a bag of canvas or heavy denim or corduroy with the above dimensions, but leave a little open space in one of the seams. Go to an aquarium-supply store and buy, for each bag you're making, ten pounds of very fine gravel, the kind that covers the bottom of fish tanks. Then fill the bag and sew up the seam tightly.

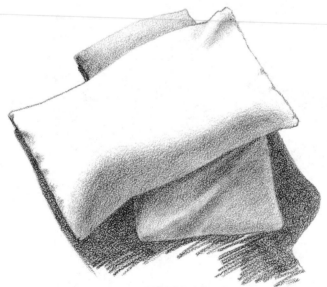

FIGURE 4.5

Yoga Mat

Yoga mats are made of a rubbery nonskid material and measure two feet by 5½ to six feet. Yoga mats are used mostly to hold your feet firmly to the floor in the standing postures. But they can also be used as padding, like for the back of your head, or to stick one body part to another, for example, the sole of your foot to the opposite inner thigh in the Tree posture.

A possible alternative is a section of the netlike rubbery material put under carpets to keep them from sliding on a wooden floor.

Chair

The best yoga chair is a metal folding chair without a padded seat. You can buy one, if you ever venture into such places, at one of those large discount stores that sell everything from soap to TVs. In this guide a yoga chair will be used mostly to get ready for sitting pranayama.

You may have a dining room or kitchen chair around the house that will serve as a suitable alternative, but be careful—if the chair is rickety, it could get broken and you might get in trouble.

Wall

Every home needs a yoga wall or at least a section of wall dedicated to yoga practice. The yoga wall is a place to brace your hands, feet, and legs. The wall or section of wall should be at least three to five feet wide and clear of furniture and all hanging decorations like plants or pictures right up to the ceiling.

Eye Bag

An eye bag, as the name suggests, is laid across the eyes during reclining pranayama or relaxation to soften and darken the eyes and so quiet the brain. Eye bags are made of cotton or silk; filled with rice, flax, or plastic pellets; and measure four inches by eight inches.

If you're handy with a needle and thread, you can easily make an eye bag. Sew a bag of some soft material with the above dimensions and fill it with something like parched rice kernels—unparched rice might attract small, unwanted visitors—or flaxseeds. You can also fill an old tube sock with rice or flax and sew up the open end.

Elastic Bandage

In the everyday world, an elastic bandage is mostly used to wrap an injured joint. Yogis, however, use the wrap to bind their head . . . a practice I'm sure you're looking forward to hearing more about (in chapter 10). Go to a drugstore and buy an elastic bandage that measures four inches wide by four feet long. We'll go into the benefits of the elastic bandage in the chapter on the Corpse posture (shavasana).

Timer

It's worthwhile to have some kind of timer for your practice. A timer helps you keep track of the length of your stay in a warm-up exercise or relaxation, the various individual stages of your breathing practice, and your entire practice. I use a digital wristwatch that has a countdown-repeat function. This means that I can set it to count down from, for example, five minutes. When the time is up and the chime sounds, the watch automatically resets itself and repeats the same countdown again and again.

You can use a kitchen timer, though it might not have the countdown-repeat function, which means you may have to periodically reset the clock. You can peek now and then at a watch without the countdown-repeat function or at a wall clock or an alarm clock, though this might be distracting and an imprecise way to track your time.

The yogis have, over the centuries, devised several ingenious ways to keep track of time. For example, there's a technique that might be called finger counting. Look at your palm. You'll see that each finger, excluding the thumb, has three sections, for a total of twelve. The yogis use the tip of the thumb to touch each of these sections in a regular pattern, over and over again, and so measure their inhales and exhales. While this is a handy way to measure, since you'll never misplace your fingers or forget to bring them to practice, and is no doubt appealing to the strict traditionalists among us, I recommend investing in a watch.

LAST WORD

This chapter is a catalogue of the kinds of props we'll use in our practice of pranayama. You might wonder, Do I really need all this stuff? Well, yes and no. Certainly it would be nice if you were properly outfitted for the journey ahead, but then again, if you have a blanket, and maybe a strap and a firm cushion, you'll be fine. You may find yourself confused about just how the props are applied, but don't worry, that will all be cleared up in later chapters. For now I'll leave you with this question-and-answer exchange, which has been making the rounds for the past few years.

> Q: How many Iyengar teachers does it take to change a lightbulb?
>
> A: Just one, but he needs a chair, a strap, three blankets, two sandbags, and a timer.

CHAPTER 5

Practice Tips

He should practice this [that is, pranayama] daily without neglect or idleness, and free from all duals (of love and hatred, and doubt and contention).

Shiva-Samhita

Practice Foundations

Pranayama practice involves much more than just the what and the how of the breaths themselves. Yoga tradition also tells us about the frequency of practice, its preferred time of day and place, the length of time of each practice, and even such seemingly unimportant information as which way to face while practicing. You will also need to have some idea about the best ways to structure your ongoing practice.

How often should I practice? Remember that one of the essential elements of pranayama practice is regularity. It would be best to practice every day of the week or at least six days a week. Of course, this is sometimes difficult or impossible. So make a commitment to be as regular as possible. At the very least, try not to miss more than two days out of every week.

When should I practice? The yogis believe that the best time to practice meditation and pranayama is just before or during sunrise, which they call the hour of Brahma (brahma-muhurta). Here the mind is calm and refreshed from the night's sleep, the atmosphere is most highly charged with prana, and the kundalini is most easily aroused. Most students do find that morning practice is best, though again, this may not always be possible. Set aside a specific period of time during the day for yourself and your practice, and try to practice at the same time every day.

Where should I practice? Dedicate a room or part of a room in your house to your practice. Make sure that the area is secure and quiet, at least during the time reserved for practice. Store your yoga props there and, if space permits, any yoga books, pictures, statues, or personal items that you find useful or inspiring.

For how long should I practice? Start your daily practice off slowly. For the first few months, spend a minimum of fifteen to twenty minutes in each session, including Corpse. Once your practice is established, you can increase the time if you wish. Some days you might want to practice more, other days less. But as I said before, commit yourself to doing something every day, if only for a few minutes. It's important to keep your practice momentum rolling, because it builds on itself, and the longer you're regular, the easier it becomes to stay regular.

But don't fiddle. It's not good enough to lie on your back in bed for an extra five minutes in the morning and concentrate on your breath. Go to your practice space, lie down with care and devotion, and breathe, even if it's only normal breathing in Corpse.

The yogis aren't solely concerned with down-to-earth practice issues like time and place. As you can read in the quote at the start of this chapter, they also want us to be in the right frame of mind for the practice, free from all duals that tug us this way and that. After all, it's pretty hard to focus on—or even care about—the subtleties of the breath if you're angry, depressed, or just plain tired.

So it's useful, at the outset of your practice, to take some time to prepare yourself mentally for the work. I have a simple opening ceremony—Purity of Direction and Homage to the Source—that gets my consciousness pointed in the right direction, so to speak.

The first thing I do is face myself toward the east, observing what the yogis call purity of direction, an integral element of all yoga practice and ritual. East, of course, is the quarter of the rising sun, the soul of the world and a symbol of the dawn of spiritual insight. Some old guides also mention facing north, the quarter of the polestar and the pinnacle of heaven.

Most old guides begin their instruction by paying homage to the founding teacher of the school, whether human or divine. Both Svatmarama and Gheranda salute, in the very first verse of their guides, the "primeval Lord" Shiva, whose teaching is compared to a "stairway" or "ladder" that helps us scale the heights of self-knowledge. Other guides pay homage to Patanjali, not only as the founder of the classical school of yoga but also as the author of famous works on Sanskrit grammar and Ayurveda, the native Indian system of medicine:

> He who removed the impurities
> Of the mind (by the teaching of yoga)
> Of speech by (his exposition of) grammar, and
> Of the body by (composing his treatise on) the science
>   of medicine, unto that doyen of sages
> I bow with joined hands.[1]

After observing purity of direction, you might like to say a few words of homage from a favorite modern guide or teacher, or words of your own devising. You could also pay tribute by simply spending a minute or two in silence, resolving to dedicate the fruits of your practice, as the yogis phrase it, to the divine.

How do I schedule daily practice? Now that I've given you my sage advice on how often to practice, what time to practice and where, how long to practice, even in which direction to aim yourself during practice, one big question remains: How do I organize and manage my practice over several months or even—if it turns out I need the time—years?

One of the more difficult things about learning something like pranayama or asana from a book is that you don't have a teacher around to help you figure out a nuts-and-bolts daily schedule and monitor your progress, adjusting your schedule as your needs and capacities change. In the old days, when the teacher and student practiced and often lived together, there was really no question about a routine and schedule. The teacher had—as we might say today—been there and done that, and knew the student inside out.

So the teacher devised the student's entire agenda, and the student simply did whatever he was told to do.

Today, of course, most of us don't have the luxury of a such close association with an experienced teacher, who can track our every move and tell us, authoritatively, what to do and when to do it. Since it isn't practical for you to move to California and live with me, the next best thing I can do is suggest a practice schedule for you.

Naturally authors of guides like this one try to be as helpful in this regard as they can. The practice schedule outlines they usually include mostly take one of two forms: either they're very specific, with fixed daily or weekly plans; or they're more open-ended, providing only a skeleton and leaving it up to you, the reader-student, to flesh out the details.

It's my feeling that the latter strategy is the more reasonable. This puts a little more responsibility on your shoulders, but in the end I think we'll all be better off. But I hope that you're acquainted with a local teacher who can give you some pointers about your practice and maybe help you tailor my generic schedule to suit your needs.

Actually all you'll really be scheduling is your timing, how slowly or quickly you progress through the program in this guide. I'll give you a general sequence of four increasingly challenging levels of practice and recommend a minimum amount of time to spend on each level.

On the first day of your first month of practice, write out your proposed schedule for that month in your journal (more on the journal in the next chapter). This way you won't have to agonize over what to practice each day. But remember that whatever you come up with isn't chiseled in granite. Be ready to change things around if the need arises. Then on the first of each following month, based on your experience in the month just passed, tune or revise your schedule as appropriate.

If you do have a regular teacher, let him know that you're practicing pranayama and that you're serious about it. Use your teacher as a resource. If you encounter particular obstacles or have questions about techniques or direction, be sure to ask him for help. It's also useful to talk with other students about their practice. Find out what's going on for them and how they're dealing with the ups and downs and the ins and outs of everyday practice. Stay alert for local classes or workshops on pranayama. While I hope this guide will help you along the way, in the end, there's no substitute for a flesh-and-blood teacher.

After you read the next chapter on the pranayama journal, you can go to appendix 1 and read over the schedule outline.

Other Tips

Students occasionally ask other questions about their breathing practice, like What should I wear? Should I practice on an empty stomach? What do I do about a stuffed-up nose? What should I do if I catch a cold?

What to wear. Wear loose-fitting clothing appropriate to the season. If you're wearing a pair of drawstring shorts, loosen the drawstring before you begin practice.

Empty stomach. We're often instructed to practice with an empty stomach, but hunger pangs can be as much of a distraction as a stuffed belly. If you're hungry before your practice, drink some milk or eat some yogurt.

Nasal wash. Sometimes it's difficult to breathe in the morning because the sinuses are congested. A nasal wash is an excellent way to open blocked air passages. It's best to buy a small pot, sometimes called a neti pot. It's made of ceramic or plastic with a long, narrow spout, and it holds about six ounces of water.

Fill the pot with warm water and a quarter teaspoon of salt. Don't forget the salt! Lean over a sink or bathtub, tilt your head to one side, and snug the spout into the higher nostril. Tip the pot up and wait. The water will flush through the sinuses and pour out the lower nostril. When the pot is empty, turn your head toward the sink and gently blow through your nose. Then fill the pot with salt water again and repeat with the head tilted to the other side.

I know that this practice may seem odd, and maybe more than a little off-putting, but trust me—once you get used to it, you'll look forward to doing it every day.

Cold. If you have a cold or flu with all its attendant miseries and afflictions—headache, stuffed nose, stiffness—you have permission to skip practice until you feel better. If you feel cold while you're practicing, warm up the room for fifteen minutes before your session or cover yourself with a blanket.

LAST WORD

Remember that your work will never proceed in a straight line. As B. K. S. Iyengar says, practice waxes and wanes like the moon. In other words, sometimes it's very strong and we go forward by leaps and bounds. Other times things seem to come to a complete standstill or even go backward. As I've mentioned, it's at these times, when we seem to be sliding back down the hill, that our commitment to the work faces its greatest test.

CHAPTER 6

Pranayama Journal

'Tis needless, the journey so hard should be.
A little turn here, another there,
And many a barrier and morass deep,
Easily surmounted will be.
I shall tell of the Way
Which at last I found,
That others in a clearer Light may See."
So I drew a chart, the best I knew,
And here it is for all
Who, wandering in forest and desert drear,
Wish that a clearer Way might revealed be.

—Franklin Merrell-Wolff,
"The Supreme Adventure," in
Pathways Through to Space:
A Personal Record of
Transformation in Consciousness

"Keep a diary," said my Teacher. "One day it will become a book. But you must write it in such a way that it should help others. People say, 'Such-and-such things did happen thousands of years ago because we read about them.' This book will be a proof that such things as are related do happen today, as they happened yesterday and will happen tomorrow—to the right people, in the right time and the right place."

—Irina Tweedie,
The Chasm of Fire

NOT ALL GUIDEBOOKS are written at the end of the road, when the traveler has returned home from the country of the Self and had time to rest and reflect on where she's been, what she's seen, and what she's learned. Some are written as the journey progresses, in the form of a journal. Reading one of these journal-guides is almost like treading the path alongside the author and sharing in all his experiences.

You don't, of course, have to be a great yogi, or even a very good writer, to keep a journal of your own practice. I started a journal soon after I began pranayama back in the early 1980s, and I've written in it, on and off, ever since. One of the requirements for my pranayama course is that all the students keep a journal of their daily work—or their lack of work. I encourage you to do the same, at least for the year or so that it takes you to work through this book.

I use my journal to keep track of where I've been and how long it's taken me to arrive at my current location; clarify and organize what I learn about myself in pranayama, including my strengths, weaknesses, and potentials; and speculate on the question Who is the breather? I also use it to determine what about my practice is useful and should be continued or adjusted, and what's not and should be dropped; inquire into how what I learn fits into and enriches my larger yoga practice and my life; exercise my imagination and creativity; and reassure myself that I'm doing as well as can be expected, considering my colossal ignorance. Keeping my journal also helps me decide where I'd like to go and avoid going in the future.

What Students Write About

The word *journal* comes from diurnal, which means "daily." Write in your journal regularly. It should be written in a special book used only for pranayama and not on loose scraps of paper stuffed into the back of desk drawers. Keep your journal handy and write as soon after your practice time as possible. Note the details of your practice session first.

Write as succinctly and objectively as possible. Avoid judgments, justifications and rationalizations, interpretations, or evaluations of your work. Don't censor your writing or worry about continuity, style, grammar, or even spelling. Listen to and write from the heart, not the head.

There's no one best way to manage a journal. Some students like to keep things simple, just a straightforward record of their daily practice. They enter the date and length of time of practice, along with an outline of the work for the day, including which exercises and breaths they performed, whether they reclined or sat (in Chair Seat or a traditional seat, which we'll go into in chapters 15 and 16), which tools they used to cultivate and refine the work, and anything else that interested them.

But other students—no doubt with more time on their hands or more enthusiastic writers—like to expand on these down-to-earth concerns. Some even embellish their writing with drawings, collages, poetry, or found objects. What do these students write about? Lots of things.

They write about how they arrived at the yoga of breathing in the first place, how the twists and turns of the road brought them to just this juncture in their journey. They write about their response to our survey of the classical and Hatha models of pranayama. They write about obstacles along the way and which assistants were useful in dealing with these obstacles. They write about their relationship with their Witness (sakshin) and the little death of Corpse (shavasana). They write about their insights into what is, and how they apply these insights to their larger yoga practice and to their life as a whole. They speculate and meditate, with the breath as their vehicle, on:

- Their feelings, thoughts, and emotions—in other words, the fluctuations—and avidya.
- The yogic life and their understanding of, and involvement with, the yamas and niyamas, either the ten (five each) outlined by Patanjali (Yoga-Sutra 2.30–45) or the twenty (ten each) listed by Svatmarama (Hatha-Yoga-Pradipika 1.16).
- The four goals of yoga.
- Their reading of other guides, both ancient and modern.
- The breath and its four qualities, and its relationship to the body and consciousness.

- Consciousness—that is, the country of the Self itself.
- The transformative power of pranayama.
- Finally, the central question that all of us must answer, Who am I?

I have the students approach this last thorny question by first asking, Who is the breather? Remember that pranayama is a tool of self-inquiry, self-transformation, and self-integration. Through the breath we can reach beyond the limits of the surface self and contact, realize, and complete our authentic self. Who is the breather? is just another way of asking, Who am I?

Some students figure out, at least to their satisfaction, their breathing identity early on and stick with it through thick and thin, with perhaps only minor modifications, as their practice progresses. Others revise their self-definition frequently, preferring to keep the question open-ended.

I would follow the lead of the latter group, at least early on in your practice. Don't jump to any conclusions about the breather's identity. Remember that it has both a physical dimension, which is fairly easy to contact, and a subtle dimension, which is trickier to expose. So start out simply and ask, Who is the breather as a body? Look at the condition and functioning of his breathing machinery. This will give you some idea about the condition and functioning of his citta, since there's no ultimate difference between the container and its contents. When you have this map in hand, then it's safe to go further.

To be honest, not all students enjoy journal writing. Some just aren't writers and have a tough time relating their breathing experiences in words. If you're not a writer, I encourage you to find other ways to record the substance and meaning of your practice. For example, you could make drawings or diagrams in your journal or record an oral journal on audiotape.

Other students claim they just can't find the time to write. After all, they've just added another practice to an already busy schedule—and now they're expected to write in a journal? My standard reply is yes! Since they're usually taking the course for credit, the time often appears as if by magic. On a typical day the journal entry shouldn't take more than ten or fifteen minutes to write, which certainly isn't a burdensome amount of time.

Then there are a few students who feel, quite honestly, that the journal is a distraction, that they can't breathe freely knowing they'll have to write about the experience later. One student wrote, "All I can think about as I'm breathing is what I'm going to say in the journal. How can I concentrate on what I'm doing?" Obviously practice comes first, and the journal should always take a backseat. If it seems like a distraction, give yourself some time, a few weeks or a month, to get comfortable with your practice and then see if it's easier to write in your journal.

LAST WORD

This is the end of the first part of our trip, although you might say that we've barely left the station. We've mostly been collecting things to take along with us, some useful information about the country of the Self, a few props to steady our way, and a journal to keep a record of our day-to-day experiences on the road. So far we haven't done a whole lot of actual practice, but that's going to change in Part Two. First, we'll meet a fellow traveler, a really nice person, then learn what many experts consider to be the most challenging of all yoga postures, next draw a map, and finally turn our attention—at last!—to the breath itself.

PART TWO
Cooperation

CHAPTER 7

The Witness

Sakshin

But to know oneself is a long process. First we must study.

—P. D. Ouspensky, *The Fourth Way*

ARE YOU READY to begin your practice of pranayama? Good. Most students are eager to set off on the journey, sitting up nice and straight, doing all sorts of curious things with their breathing rhythms, maybe using their fingers to block one or both of their nostrils, holding their breath for X number of counts. All of this will certainly be possible for you one day . . . but not today, and not for a good while to come. As I cautioned you in the introduction, this guide follows what I call the lions, elephants, and tigers approach to pranayama.

With any trip you take, you first have to get yourself ready. There are a lot of big and small details to look after before you can go: packing, putting your mail and the paper on hold, arranging for your neighbors to look after the houseplants and the cat, and so on. That's sort of what we'll be doing in Part Two of the guide, beginning with this chapter.

There's something that you must do before you trek into the country of the Self that you usually don't have to do before an everyday trip—and that's get some information about yourself. In the country of the Self, it's not enough just to know where you're going and how to get there; you also have to know something about who is going. Students who leave in a hurry, especially without the guiding hand of an experienced teacher, without taking the time to survey themselves, often find themselves struggling or, worse, getting completely lost.

You might think that, to do this, it's time to roll up our sleeves and get to work on some of those movement and breathing exercises

71

we're always reading about in books and magazines. Not so fast, again. The lions, elephants, and tigers approach insists that if you want to change something about yourself—whether it's your body, your breath, or your consciousness—you first have to establish what is.

So our first task is not to do something or change something or make any effort at all. Just the opposite. We're not going to do anything but simply observe and acquaint ourselves with our everyday body and breath and find out what is. I know this goes against the grain of some students, who wonder how they can fix the problem and change themselves without doing something. But remember (from chapter 2) that doing nothing, the natural and nondeliberate stopping of the breath, called kevala-kumbhaka, is the goal of pranayama itself. I think it's appropriate that we begin our practice in the same way. We do nothing but observe the what is. Without this basic awareness, any breathing exercises we try aren't likely to be much help.

We'll need a friend to help us with this task, someone who can stand back from and contemplate our what is, without judgment or expectation. The yogis call this friend the Witness (sakshin). It'll help us take our first few steps on our journey and then stay by our side for every step thereafter.

So where do you find a Witness? To answer this question, let's study our own everyday consciousness (citta) for a moment. You may remember that it's forever in movement or fluctuation. These fluctuations—induced by perceptions, thoughts, emotions, memories, or whatever—are the contents of citta. Because of avidya, we forget our authentic self and identify solely with these contents, imagining—wrongly—that they define and limit who we are. This results in the bad axle hole (duhkha), suffering.

But while we're habitually forgetful and identified solely with the contents, there's no absolute necessity that we be this way—otherwise, liberation would be impossible. We can, at any time, remember ourselves and disidentify with this "unsteady flux," as Sri Aurobindo calls it, and simply consider all this ferment "as the Witness seated above the surge of the forces of Nature."[1]

For most of us, this represents an entirely new way of looking at the world and ourselves. All our life we're taught to assign values to people and things, to analyze and criticize, but rarely to accept and simply mirror what is. The Witness engages the outer and inner worlds on their own terms and lets them speak in their own words. It's present-centered, with no memories of the past or concerns about the future; self-reliant, independent of the approval or disapproval of others; and self-accepting, in both success and failure.

PRACTICE

You might imagine that befriending your Witness is difficult, but it's really not. The Witness is accessible at any time to anyone, with no special training, except if you want to continue witnessing while asleep.

We'll start to work with our Witness in earnest in the next chapter, but for now here's a simple exercise to get you started. Begin with what's most palpable about yourself, your body. Sit back in your chair or lie down on the floor and close your eyes. Step back from your body, as you might step back from an intriguing puzzle or unfamiliar object, and slowly scan your awareness over its surface. You can do this methodically from feet to head. Feel, for example, where your skin comes into contact with the world, the border between what's inside and what's outside, or where your skin is soft or stretched over bones, or where it's warm or cool or cold. Alternatively you can just allow your Witness to play over your body wherever it wants to go.

Be sure to include in your scan all those areas of the body where we don't often go with awareness, especially the back body (we'll do an exercise to contact the back body in chapter 9 and in appendix 2). Also be sure to notice which areas, if any, are beyond the ken of your Witness. Somewhere along the way, you may have lost large tracts of yourself to a kind of physical avidya. Your Witness will one day help you to enlighten these dark areas.

Then direct your awareness inward, away from the surface, toward the contents of your citta. What do you see in there? As I've said, we ordinarily identify with the fluctuations and so submerge and lose ourselves in them. But we don't have to. Step back now from the contents of your citta and regard what you see from sundry angles, without favoring any one of them. Appreciate that you can remember yourself and disidentify yourself from the fluctuations, allow them expression without getting mixed up in them. While they may be a part of you, they're ultimately not all of you.

HOW IT HELPS

The Witness is the means to inquire into and enlighten our breathing machinery and breathing behavior, the what is, and so prepare for formal pranayama. When my beginning breathers introduce the Witness into their practice, they generally learn two important things about themselves as breathers: Just as they don't know their authentic self because of avidya, neither do they know their authentic breather, and they're unconsciously doing something to their authentic breath that they don't need to do or shouldn't be doing.

They also learn that this very elementary act of witnessing, and not doing anything, is enough to initiate the process of transformation, both physical and mental. When the Witness shines a light on the unnecessary or unhealthy doing-somethings of the surface self and surface breather, they immediately lose some of their potency, and the grip of avidya, and so suffering, is weakened. Stubborn tensions spontaneously dissolve and the everyday breath is effortlessly controlled (ayama). When this happens, our breathing subtly changes, and we get a taste of the authentic breath. As one student wrote, breathing "just happens."

GOING FURTHER

While our Witness is easy enough to contact, the real challenge is to stay in contact for more than a few seconds. The link to our new traveling companion is necessarily weak at first, and so it's not surprising that we quickly slip back into the vritti-stream and forget all about it—and ourselves. Don't be too concerned if this happens to you early on. With regular practice your link to the Witness will be strengthened until, at some point, its presence in your life will be almost constant and effortless.

You may discover, as many of my students do, that the fluctuations themselves don't especially like being witnessed and brought into the light of day. Witnessing tends to diminish the hold that this mind-stream has on us, and like any living being, it battles to survive

and fulfill its life's role . . . which is to keep us forgetful and in ignorance. You'll need to be patient and persevere. Developing your Witness is like developing a muscle: the more you exercise it, the
stronger it gets.

Always check in with your Witness at the start of practice, both
asana and pranayama. Take a few minutes to look at your fluctuations for that day. Notice how you're feeling, about yourself, your
practice, about life in general. Are any obstacles looming on the
horizon? If there are, just witness them, nothing more. The Witness not only sees but also, as it gains in strength and experience,
suggests possible courses of action. Be sure to listen carefully for
any words of wisdom from your Witness.

PLAYING AROUND: THE WITNESS

Once you've established a good working relationship with your Witness in formal practice, then bring it into your everyday life. Play
around with it as much as possible, regularly or randomly, during
the day. Of course, it's not easy to remember to do this at first. So I
carry around a memory aid, what I call a remembrancer (which means
"one who causes another to remember something"), something odd
or out of the ordinary, like a small stone or a ring on an ordinarily
unringed finger, that reminds me about my Witness every time I
touch it or see it. Just remember that the remembrancer will eventually get stale, and so you'll need to find a different one periodically.

LAST WORD

The Witness really helps you to do two things: remember yourself
and ask Who am I?; and study yourself, look at specific things about
yourself, including your breath.

Like Patanjali's purusha, the Witness is the pure light of our consciousness, who sees the contents but who can't be seen itself. It's
often compared to a spectator at a play who sits quietly in the audi-
ence, thoroughly enjoying the performance, whether it's drama or
comedy, but not itself participating. The Witness transcends, or
climbs above, the relatively narrow confines of the surface self and
reflects the contents of citta but is never attracted to (raga) or repelled

by (dvesha) anything that passes before it on the stage. It's in us "merely as an onlooker (sakshin) who in all cognition, present as its innermost nucleus looks on at worldly action and at its illusions without being in the least mixed up in it."[2]

CHAPTER 8

Corpse
Introduction to Shavasana

This thing called "corpse" we dread so much is living with us here and now.

—Milarepa, *The Tibetan Book of Living and Dying*

NOW THAT YOU'VE made the acquaintance of your Witness, let's put your new friend to work. This chapter and the two that follow are a kind of minicourse in the posture known as shavasana, which is usually translated as the "Corpse posture."

Corpse seems like an odd name for a yoga posture. In fact, some teachers prefer to call it something else—as, for example, the Sponge—or refer to it rather tamely as the relaxation pose. They fear, perhaps with good reason, that our usual associations with the word corpse will cool our desire to practice the posture. But there are very good reasons for naming this posture Corpse.

You may already have some experience with Corpse. It's commonly used as a well-deserved rest, both physically and psychologically, at the end of an asana session, though some schools of yoga make regular, repeated use of Corpse as a kind of way station between postures during the session. The label is appropriate, of course, because we're asked to lie completely still on our back and emulate, at least outwardly, a lifeless body. But inwardly our Witness is still very much alive and kicking, doing its job of closely monitoring the body-mind.

Years ago I had a teacher who would holler at anyone in class rash enough to stir in any way during Corpse, even if our nose was itching like crazy and we absolutely had to scratch. "Stop that moving," he would shout out, and the culprit would get quiet again in a hurry. Rest assured I won't do the same to you, but understand that stillness, both physical and mental, is the essence of the posture. Without it, it's difficult to calm the fluctuations and achieve true relaxation.

Corpse is also so named because of its symbolic significance. You may know that the yogis, like many other Easterners, believe that after the death of our physical body, the authentic self will eventually come back to life in another body. "As a man casts off his worn-out clothes and takes on other new ones," relates Krishna to Arjuna, "so does the embodied self cast off its worn-out bodies and enters other new ones."[1] You may think, "Great, I get another chance," but the yogis don't see it that way. They declare that the endless round of unenlightened existence brings nothing but sorrow in its wake.

So the yogis in effect beat death at its own game by symbolically dying, not once but twice. The first death occurs at the outset of the journey into the country of the Self, when the aspirant is initiated by her guru or spiritual preceptor. The Sanskrit word for initiation or dedication, diksha, is rooted in a verb that means "to cut" or "to destroy." Through initiation, then, the aspirant cuts her attachment and so figuratively dies to her worldly life, while she dedicates herself to new ways of thinking and acting and the cessation of all sorrow—and rebirth—in self-liberation. But initiation is only the first step. Without it liberation is nearly impossible, at least according to tradition, though even with it there's no assurance of reaching the final destination.

The second symbolic death coincides with the moment of liberation. As long as we cling to life (abhinivesha) and our mistaken belief in our own separateness (asmita), with its attendant likes (raga) and dislikes (dvesha), we'll surely die one day, only to return again to much the same state of affairs. But as soon as we give up this clinging and sense of isolation, we die forever, but now to both our ignorance (avidya) and the cycle of physical death and rebirth. The Corpse posture is a kind of rehearsal for these symbolic deaths, a little death at the end of every practice session, at once a self-initiation and self-surrender.

Incidentally if you object to calling this posture Corpse, then you might instead use Gheranda's name for it, *mritasana*, which means the "Death posture."

PRELIMINARY

Before reading the next sections, lie down in Corpse for about ten minutes (assuming that you already have some training with this posture). Then ask yourself the following questions:

- How do I prepare for Corpse? What props, if any, do I use?
- Is my Witness present when I practice Corpse?
- What kinds of adjustments, if any, do I make in this posture?
- How do I occupy myself while I'm in Corpse? What do I think about or not think about?
- When I'm finished, how do I leave the posture?
- Finally, how do I feel about Corpse? Is it a posture that I enjoy and practice regularly, or is it uncomfortable and something I avoid?

Write down your answers to these questions in your journal to give yourself a picture of the what is of your everyday Corpse.

You may not be accustomed to preparing for Corpse with a lot of detailed adjustments. After all, what's so hard about lying down supine on the floor? Nothing really . . . but remember that Corpse isn't simply racking out for a few minutes and napping. Believe it or not, some yoga authorities assert that it's one of the most difficult of all the yoga asanas to perform successfully.

I've been taught over the years to be very diligent about how I organize myself for and then maintain the posture. If the essence of Corpse is stillness, then its cornerstone is physical balance, which in turn leads to the ultimate state of mental balance or equanimity (samatva). A student once asked one of my teachers what Corpse is supposed to feel like. He paused for a moment—no doubt for dramatic effect—and then replied, "Nothing." We all laughed, but he was serious. When skillfully executed, Corpse conduces to a neutral state that, as Patanjali remarks about asana in general, relaxes all physical tension and expands our normally limited consciousness to coincide with the infinite (ananta).

Creating this balance is a tricky tightrope-walking feat for most beginners, even in a position as ostensibly uncomplicated as Corpse.

Almost every body is more or less crooked somewhere and somehow, and over time we tend to get habituated to our crookedness. This becomes a kind of false neutral, which we naturally assume every time we repose in Corpse. We imagine that we're lying in balance, but actually our head is turned to one side, our shoulders are skewed, one side of our torso is shorter than the other, our legs and arms aren't angled evenly on the floor—the list goes on and on.

Though we're not overtly aware of our crookedness, somewhere in the recesses of our consciousness, we do feel it. It generates tension and the bane of Corpse—and for that matter, all of yoga practice—the dreaded fluctuations. Then we feel compelled to wiggle and waggle to relieve the tension and calm the fluctuations, which then provokes even more fluctuating, and so on it goes. How do we end up so crooked? Life just makes us that way. Handedness and footedness (if there's such a word), unhealthy postural habits, injuries, emotional upsets, and daily stress—all of this and more contributes to crookedness. My students report all kinds of interesting and quirky crookedness in their bodies.

You can easily check on your own crookedness. Lie down in your everyday Corpse and make your best adjustments. For a few minutes witness the back of your head, torso, and limbs, using the floor as a tactile aid to contact the back body. What do you feel, if anything? Pay special attention to how the heels, sacrum, shoulder blades, knuckles, and head are sitting on the floor. First survey the left side, then the right (reverse if you're left-handed), and finally compare the two sides. What do you discover? Be sure to store this information away in your memory or write about it in your journal.

So what do we do about crookedness? The first step, of course, which by now you've begun to discover, is to get clear about the what is. Where and how are you crooked? Sometimes, although you are working at it, it's difficult to answer this by yourself, just because you're so conditioned to what is. You might want to get the help of a yoga friend or teacher to help you clarify your crookedness, through both touch and description. Then you can begin to adjust whatever's crooked. I'll give you some tips on how to do this later and in chapters to come.

Beginners in Corpse often respond to my expert corrections with an incredulous, "Are you sure I'm straight?" There's a chance that your newfound balance in Corpse will make you feel crooked and not a little uncomfortable. There's also a chance that, unconsciously reacting to this discomfort, you'll shift back to what feels right and make yourself comfortable—and crooked—again. Don't worry. It'll take some time before you get balanced, and then comfortable being in balance, but with practice almost everybody can establish at least a fair approximation of neutrality, though some students are permanently thrown off balance by things like physical disabilities or scoliosis.

Mapping the Body

In this guide we'll also use Corpse—with the assistance of our Witness—to gather material about ourselves with which we'll begin to map out the country of the Self (in chapter 9). What kind of map will this be? I'm sure you'll agree that it's a good idea, before leaving on a trip to any new place, to study a map. A map gives us an overall picture of the city or country we'll be visiting, shows us directions, points of interest and what to avoid, the distances between things. Of course, we can't go down to the corner cartographical supply store to buy this kind of map, so we'll have to draw it ourselves.

Our map will include both surface features—the lay of our body's land, so to speak—and the hidden inner space of the body. You may wonder, Isn't my body stuffed with bones and organs and whatnot like a Thanksgiving turkey? Where's my inner space, and why do I need to find it?

Actually you're right, there's no real inner space in your body. As with many other places we go in yoga, our inner space exists only in our imagination. Most of us know at least some things about our outer body—even if it's only where our arms and legs are—but very little about the inner body. But without an appreciation of the fullness of our inner space, our own three-dimensionality, we tend to perceive ourselves as flat, one-dimensional creatures, like cardboard cutouts. Our breath then penetrates into only a very limited area of our body, usually the front torso, and the remainder is left untouched and unbreathed. Awareness of our inner space, with its axis at our front spine, helps us to further calm the body and realize our authentic breather. (We'll go into this in greater detail in chapter 9.)

Yogis are indefatigable mapmakers, both of the world around them and of their own bodies. As a matter of fact, we all are, though we're not usually awake to what we're up to because our maps, and our mapmaking, are so much a part of what we do. But if we didn't make these kinds of maps of the world around us, routine outings to the corner market or yoga class would take a lot more time and effort.

It's much the same with our body map. Just as the old mapmakers drew their maps after exploring and surveying uncharted lands, so also we draw our body map by moving through the world and letting the world rub up against our body. Without movement and tactile experience, we wouldn't be able to construct a body map at all, or at least our map would be rather hazy.

Ideally, when this map conforms in large measure to the actual topography of our body, we move through the world with assurance, grace, intelligence, and joy. But this ideal is rarely realized, and our map is often haphazardly drawn or even seriously distorted. Whatever we do, then, including breathing, is adversely affected. We wind up confused and lost, asking for directions. Happily we all have the capacity to erase and then redraw the map, and however bewildered we may be now, we always have the opportunity to find ourselves again.

This is one reason why it's important to stay still in Corpse. To a large extent, we all draw our body maps based on information gathered through movement and effort. There's nothing inherently wrong with this. Without activity our map is incomplete, and so we're poorly oriented toward our own body and don't feel ourselves to be completely alive.

The problem is that many of us become less mobile and more sedentary over the years, shrinking our maps considerably. Consciously or unconsciously, we confine ourselves to a very small range of movement when, as the yogis clearly demonstrate, our movement potential is vast. By keeping quiet in Corpse, we can, for a time, wipe the slate clean and dissolve some of the habitual restrictions we unconsciously impose on ourselves and our movements. Then we can, by re-creating this rediscovered sense of spaciousness in our practice, begin to redraw our map.

HOW IT HELPS

Svatmarama relates that lying in Corpse "removes tiredness and enables the mind (and whole body) to relax."[2] Another way to use Corpse is to spend a few minutes in the posture at the start of your asana or pranayama practice to gather your thoughts and rehearse the sequence of postures or breathing techniques in your imagination.

Beginning students often underestimate the value of rest at the end of their practice and so either skimp on the time spent in Corpse or skip it altogether. But it's important to remember that the unceasing rhythmic alteration of work and rest pervades all of life, and these elements are the two great wings of yoga practice that must continuously temper and balance each other.

Mapping the body, as a preparation for our expedition, helps us define who and where and how we are. Like all maps, a body map gives us the means to locate and orient ourselves in space and navigate through our world with skill and grace. With it, too, we can better interpret and integrate our perceptions and experiences, stimulate and intensify our imagination, to add detail or color to our known world, and charge our interest in and enthusiasm for traveling beyond fixed borders. We begin to see the territory in new and startling ways, which alerts us to the many possibilities of a more spacious life beyond our limited what is. Our body map will establish a framework for both our reclining and sitting practice and contribute to the liberation of our authentic breather.

GOING FURTHER

Be sure to practice Corpse regularly, not only after a formal practice session but for a few minutes at a time throughout your day, especially after a hard day at work (and aren't they all hard?).

PLAYING AROUND: BODY MAP

Keep your body map in mind as you go about your daily business. With the help of your Witness, watch how the "what is" you define in Corpse manifests in other positions, like sitting or standing or walking down the street. Keep your body map up to date by writing about it, or drawing actual maps, in your journal.

LAST WORD

In the next chapter we'll conduct our initial mapping expedition into the country of the Self. This will be an atypical expedition, surely, since we won't actually be going anywhere, just lying on our back in Corpse. But I can almost guarantee you that there will be some of the excitement of a real wilderness trek, as we learn some interesting things about ourselves. And maybe, depending on the weather and any unforeseen obstacles, there will be some of the discomfort, too.

We'll take as our area of exploration here what the yogis call the "gross body." Now before you take offense, I'm not suggesting that your body is gross, at least as we understand the popular usage of that word. Instead, "gross body" is an English rendering of the Sanskrit phrase sthula-sharira, which the yogis use to signify our physical frame. Another name for this body is the food sheath (anna-maya-kosha), though thinking of our body as food might seem a little gross. Whatever you call it, it's a vehicle for the subtler bodies the yogis have infiltrated during their own mapping voyages. Then in chapter 10 we'll work with our five traditional senses—skin, eyes, nose, tongue, and ears—in Corpse.

CHAPTER 9

Mapping the "Gross Body" in Corpse

Each of us has the right to speak of his coastline, his mountains, his deserts, none of which conforms to those of another. Individually we are obligated to make a map of our own homeland, our own field or meadow. We carry engraved in our hearts the map of the world as we know it.

Gazing at the map, I begin to see a portrait of myself. All the diversity of the world is intimated on the parchment, even as this diversity is intimated within me. An aura of remoteness hovers about its contours, as it does about my head, clarifying what I see. Both the map and myself cling to the invisibility of what we represent. Nor is the tension between us that of myself and it, but of the merging of these. The map and myself are the same.

—James Cowan, *A Mapmaker's Dream*

NOWADAYS MAPS are made with computers based on information gathered by earth-orbiting satellites. In the old days, though, intrepid explorers ventured out into unknown territory with their trusty instruments to make their measurements of the land up close and personal—at least this is the way I like to imagine it happened. That's sort of what we'll be doing, too, for our body map. No satellites for us.

I can't really say what your map will look like, but it's unlikely you'll ever really finish drawing it. It's better to think of it as a perpetual work in progress, changing both in its general outlines and in its specific details as you yourself venture more deeply into the country of the Self. Don't be surprised either—or discouraged—if one day you realize that your map is outdated and that you need to start it all over again. Drawing and then discarding maps is just part of the business of answering the question Who am I?

There are six general areas that we'll be mapping in this chapter: the feet and legs, including the head of the thighbone; the sacrum, tailbone, pubis, and hip points, all structures of the pelvis; the rib case; the shoulder yoke (a word, by the way, with the same root as yoga), made up of the shoulder blades, collarbones, and breastbone; the spine; and the neck and head.

PRELIMINARY

First, read through all the instructions that follow and gather up any props you think you might need before you start. Make sure you won't be disturbed in any way for however long you decide to conduct your mapping operation. Lie on your back on the floor, which may be bare or padded with a folded blanket or sticky mat, but not a soft mattress. Close your eyes. If you wear glasses, take them off. If your head doesn't rest comfortably on the floor, support your neck with a firmly rolled blanket or towel.

Cover your eyes with an eye bag or use an elastic bandage to wrap your head and eyes (see the Six-Openings Seal, in chapter 10). If you use the wrap, though, it's best to remove your contact lenses if you wear them. Whenever you practice Corpse, always lie parallel and perpendicular, not angled, to the walls of your room.

Then contact your Witness. For the first few times you strike out into the country of the Self, your Witness may seem a bit disinterested in the proceedings and periodically wander off into the woods, leaving you lost and bewildered. As soon as you realize you're alone, call your friend back. If you have trouble holding on to your Witness, try setting the countdown-repeat function on a digital wristwatch to three or four minutes, and use its regular beeping as an auditory cue. As you return again and again to your mapping work, your Witness will slowly become a more interested participant.

In traditional Corpse the legs are laid flat on the floor, with the heels a few inches apart. In this chapter and the following, I'd like to use a modified Corpse position, with the knees bent and supported in one of two ways.

Bent-Knee Corpse

PRACTICE: BENT-KNEE CORPSE 1

In this first variation, the bent legs are held in place with a strap.

Lie on your back and slip a widely looped strap over your legs and up onto your pelvis. Don't do anything with it yet; just lay it loosely across your body and on the floor. Bend your knees to approximate right angles with your soles on the floor, thighs parallel to each other. Rest your fingertips on your inner thighs, just to either side of the pubic bone. Right below your fingertips, about a hand's width apart, are the ball-shaped heads of your thighbones (femurs), which nestle in the cup-shaped hip sockets (acetabula).

Exhale and lift your right foot away from the floor until the thigh is perpendicular to the floor. Imagine there's a long pencil attached to your kneecap with its point touching the ceiling. Begin to draw a large circle on the ceiling, rotating the thigh first clockwise for a few turns, then counterclockwise for an equal number of turns. Gradually diminish the circumference of this circle until your thigh comes to a stop. Now the femur head is centered directly in the hip socket. Allow the bony ball to sink through the socket to the back of your pelvis and, with an exhale, release the foot back onto the floor. Repeat with the left leg.

When you have a feel for the centered femur heads, slip the strap up your thighs to just above the knees and tighten it, securing the thighs parallel to each other. Make sure that you don't allow the thighs to press heavily out against the strap—that tends to harden the groins. Turn your feet inward, pigeon-toe-like, so that your heels are farther apart than your big toes. (see fig. 9.1).

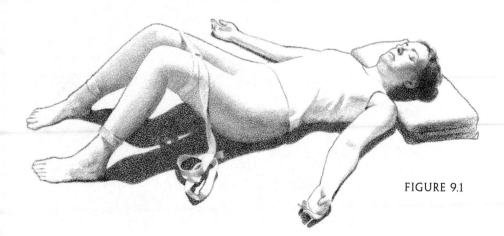

FIGURE 9.1

PRACTICE: BENT-KNEE CORPSE 2

In this second variation of Bent-Knee Corpse, the knees are supported by a bolster, which can be of any thickness. Some students prefer a thick round bolster, others a thinly rolled blanket. You can use a firm round bolster or one or more rolled-up blankets, and optionally two sandbags.

First, learn to center the femur heads in the hip sockets, as described in variation 1. Then rest your bent knees over a bolster. Experiment with the thickness of the bolster until you find one to your liking. Let your feet turn out evenly to the sides. If you have difficulty relaxing your groins, lay a sandbag across the top of each thigh, parallel to the crease of the groin. The two bags should form a V, with its apex near the pubis. Pile on as much weight as you have, if you have more than two bags, but be sure to weigh both thighs down equally. Then release the thighs away from the Sandbags (see fig. 9.2).

HOW IT HELPS

Neither of these Corpse versions is better than the other, but some students prefer to use the weight of their thighbones to release and deepen the groins, while others want to take it easier and use the weight of the sandbags. Experiment with both versions. You may find one you prefer, or you may continue to work with both for different effects.

It's very important, whether reclining or sitting (or standing, for that matter), to first center the femur heads and soften the groins, an

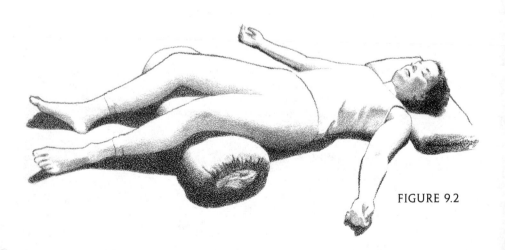

FIGURE 9.2

action that initiates a chain of spontaneous reactions, which lengthen the spine, ground the legs, and deepen the space of the breath.

Be sure to work with this centering action not only in Bent-Knee Corpse but in your other asanas as well.

GOING FURTHER

For now we'll be working in Bent-Knee Corpse. Eventually, though, you'll have to decide, for your everyday Corpse, if you want to continue to use the bent-knee variation or straighten your legs in the traditional manner. If you want to do the latter, always start from the bent-knee position and center the femur heads first. Then, one at a time, each time with an exhale, push out from the hip through the leg and slide the heel along the floor until the knee is straight and the leg is on the floor. Imagine that you're lengthening along the back of the leg. Then soften the groin and let the leg turn out.

Make sure that the heels are resting evenly on the floor. It's common for one foot to be angled slightly differently than the other. This is usually caused by stickiness in the hip joint, not the ankle. Twist that leg back and forth a few times like a windshield wiper to help release the hip.

Pelvis: Sacrum and Coccyx, Pubis, Hip Points

The pelvis is shaped like a basin. (At least that's what some old anatomist once thought, since that's what the Latin word pelvis means.) It's a funny-looking basin, though—you could swear that somebody took a big bite out of one side and punched a big hole in the bottom. There are several important landmarks located on the pelvis that we'll need to know about for our mapping expedition.

The back of the pelvis (and the base of the spine) is the sacrum. Its anatomical name is os sacrum, another Latin term that means "sacred or holy bone." I read somewhere once that the sacrum got its name because, according to one Western legend, it doesn't decay after the death of the body and so is the seat of our resurrection. Made of five fused vertebrae and shaped like a downward-pointing triangle (when your torso is upright), the sacrum is the back wall of the pelvis and the base of the flexible part of the spine.

At the very tip or apex of the sacrum is the vestigial tailbone, the coccyx. It must once have reminded some imaginative anatomist of a hooked bird's beak, because coccyx is from a Greek word that means "cuckoo."

The pubis is one of the three parts of the hipbone, along with the ilium and the ischium. It's located at the front base of the pelvis, where the two branches of the hipbones join together.

The hip points mark the front ends of the top rim or crest of the pelvis. You can find them six or so inches to either side of the navel (see fig. 9.3).

PRACTICE

Find the two hip points and press your middle fingers against these knobs. Reach your thumbs around to the back of the pelvis and burrow them into the two dimples that mark the ends of the top, or what's technically called the base, of the sacrum. Spread the buttocks away from the sacrum, so that the bone rests broadly and evenly on the floor.

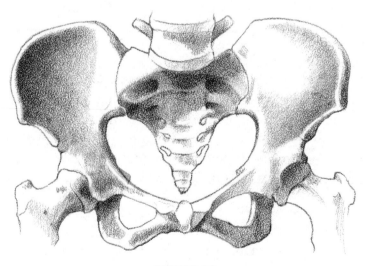

FIGURE 9.3

Push your feet lightly against the floor and funnel the back of the pelvis toward your tail. Imagine that your tail is stretching out to your heels like a long monkey tail. Watch your lower back release toward but not flatten on the floor. Pull the dimples of the sacrum apart, widening the back of the pelvis. At the same time, push the hip points toward each other and the navel, narrowing the front of the pelvis. Imagine that the sacrum is lifting lightly away from the floor into your pelvis.

Then rest the fingertips lightly on the hip points. How much space is there between the fingers and the floor? Take a few slow, full breaths. Watch the fingers open and close with the inhales and exhales.

Slide your fingertips down into and along the creases of the front groins. Poke gently around for the pubis at the front base of the pelvis. Press your fingertips on the ends of this bone where it joins the inner thighs. Press the ends of the bone toward its midline. Like the two hip points, the two branches of the pubis should narrow.

How much space is there between the pubis and sacrum? The bottom of the pelvis is quite narrow, but can you sense this area at the bottom of your pelvis at the perineum? There's a muscular diaphragm at the bottom of the pelvis that, like the thoracic diaphragm, expands and contracts with the inhales and exhales. Take a couple of minutes to breathe into the bottom of your pelvis.

While the sacrum is securely ligatured between the wings (alae) of the pelvis, it does have a little play, called nutation or nodding. On the inhale the sacrum rocks backward, on the exhale forward. This induces a rhythmic pulse at the base of the spine that pumps the fluid circulating in the spinal canal and skull.

Let's purposely exaggerate the nodding of the sacrum. Slowly inhale and press your lower back down against the floor, then slowly exhale and arch it off the floor again. Continue for a few minutes, flattening and arching the back, and so nodding the sacrum, in rhythm with your breath. You might also want to reverse the movements with the breath, arching on the inhale and flattening on the exhale.

HOW IT HELPS

These actions soften the muscles of the buttocks, outer hips, and lower back. This, in turn, helps balance the pelvis on the heads of the femurs and ground the back and elevate the front spine (more on the back and front spine later in the chapter). All of this contributes to a steady and comfortable position, whether reclining or sitting. These actions also play an important role in the Lower Belly Lock (see chapter 20).

Caution. Be sure not to press too hard on the pubis or tuck the coccyx and flatten the lower spine. We want to lengthen the lumbar and soften the lumbar muscles, but never flatten the natural inward curve (lordosis) of this area of the spine.

Rib Case

There are twelve pairs of bow-shaped ribs. The heads of all the ribs attach through joints to the twelve thoracic vertebrae. The top seven pairs of ribs attach directly to the sternum in the front (and are called true ribs), rib pairs eight through ten attach indirectly to the sternum through the cartilages of the higher ribs (and so are called false ribs. The two lowest pairs, fittingly called the floating ribs, have no connection to the sternum (see fig. 9.4).

The rib case supports the thorax, which would simply collapse in on itself without these semirigid stays, and protects the heart and lungs. Though we're not usually aware of it, the ribs are in constant movement through three dimensions as we breathe—out and in, up and down, and forward and back. They do this by rotating in their joints in the thoracic spine with the help of the breathing muscles like the intercostals and the scalenes. Without this movement breathing would be impossible. Because of old injuries, habitual physical misalignment, or chronic emotional distress, many people have rigid ribs, which greatly interferes with their breathing.

The breathing movement of the ribs is often illustrated by the bucket handle model. Imagine a bucket lying on its side. A line drawn between the two ears—the handle attachments (and yes, they're really called that)—is parallel to the floor, and the top of the C-shaped handle is resting on, and so forming a forty-five-degree angle with, the floor. The bucket handle, of course, stands in for any one pair or all twelve pairs of ribs, though the lower ribs tend to move more than the upper and so fit this model better. The two ears stand for the rib pairs' attachments to the sides of the spine, so in this model the spine itself is perpendicular to the floor. The sternum is located at the top of the curved handle.

On the inhale the handle slowly lifts until it is parallel to the floor (see fig. 9.5a). Then on the exhale it slowly returns to the floor (see fig. 9.5b). Of course, the model isn't perfect. The bucket handle doesn't expand and contract in three dimensions as it lifts and descends . . . but you get the idea.

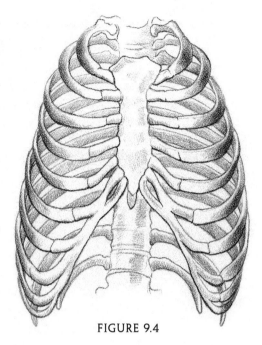

FIGURE 9.4

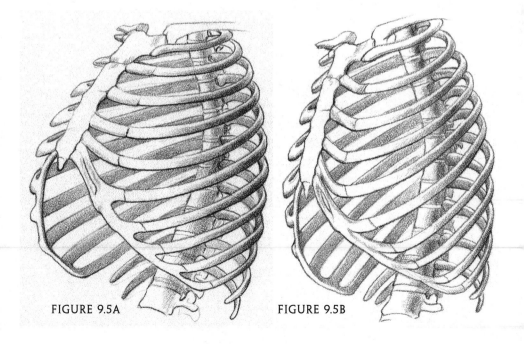

FIGURE 9.5A

FIGURE 9.5B

PRACTICE

It's difficult to get a precise feel for the breathing movements of the rib roots on your own. Our sense of the back body is typically dull or nonexistent, but eventually we'll need to bring the back into the full light of consciousness. If you can find a yoga partner, or just someone with a friendly pair of hands, you might try the back body exercise in appendix 2.

In the meantime take a few minutes to watch how the ribs move as you breathe, using the floor as a tactile aid for the back body. Lay your hands on your front ribs, starting with the lower ones, and slowly move up toward the shoulders or out toward the armpits, crossing your arms in front of your torso to reach each hand to the opposite side. Spend as much time as you like at each level.

On the inhales balloon the ribs and fill your palms. On the exhales press the ribs slowly down and in. Can you get a sense of the ever-changing shape of your thorax? How deep is it? How wide? How long? Breathe equally into both the front and back torso.

HOW IT HELPS

This exercise helps increase awareness of the back torso, the inner space of the thorax, and the breathing movements of the ribs as they rotate in their spinal roots.

Shoulders: Shoulder Blades, Collarbones, Breastbone

The shoulder yoke includes the two collarbones (clavicles) and the two shoulder blades (scapulas). For convenience I'm including the breastbone (sternum) in this section, though technically it's part of the rib case. The yoke hangs by muscles from the base of the skull and sits on the top of the sternum, at the attachment of the two collarbones.

Each scapula is shaped like a right triangle. The two right-angled legs of the triangle define the upper (or superior) and the inner (or medial) borders, which parallel the lines of the shoulder and the spine, respectively. The hypotenuse of this right triangle is called the lateral border. The scapulas are very mobile and can move up and down the back, and away from and toward the spine.

Each clavicle looks like an old-fashioned key, a roughly S-shaped bone that connects the top of the sternum to a bony projection of the scapula, the acromion, which you can feel as a small bump on the top of your shoulder near the shoulder joint. Together the two clavicles help maintain the breadth of the upper chest.

Sternum comes from a word that means "to spread out." The bone has three parts, which are called, from top to bottom, the manubrium or handle, just below the hollow of the throat; the body; and the xiphoid, which means "sword," just above the soft upper abdomen. You can picture the sternum as a knife with a broad blade, its tip pointing toward the navel and its handle at the throat (see fig. 9.4).

PRACTICE

For this practice you might need two folded blankets or towels and two sandbags. Lift your pelvis a few inches off the floor, so that the weight of the torso presses the scapulas firmly against the floor, which, in turn, presses the scapulas firmly against the back. Push your feet against the floor, so the scapulas, like the sacrum, are scrubbed down the back toward the tail. Hold for a few breaths, then on an exhale slowly roll your lower back and pelvis onto the floor.

Reach your arms straight up toward the ceiling, palms facing each other. Rock slightly from side to side and spread the back ribs away from the spine. Imagine that your arms are rooted not in the shoulder joints, where the upper arm bones are cupped in the shoulder blades, but much farther back, in the inner borders of the shoulder blades. Without narrowing the back between the shoulder blades, return your arms slowly to the floor (see fig. 9.6).

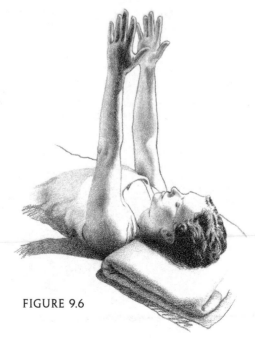

FIGURE 9.6

Then touch your fingertips to the fronts of the shoulders and lengthen the backs of the upper arms away from the torso (see fig. 9.7). Push out from your inner scapulas through your elbows. Lay the forearms on the floor and angle the arms away from the torso somewhere between thirty and forty-five degrees. Turn the arms outward from the inner scapulas, as you slide these bones down your back. Rest the backs of the hands on the floor near the index-finger knuckles. Heavily release the heads of the upper arm bones (humeri) downward, toward the floor. Relax the thumbs.

If you're tighter in the shoulders and armpits, you may have trouble getting comfortable with your hands and arms flat on the floor. You can then:

- Lay a sandbag across each of your wrists or across your wrists and palms; if you do the latter, be sure the bag weighs down most heavily on the mound of the thumb (see fig. 9.8a).

- Lift the backs of your hands and wrists a few inches off the floor on folded blankets or towels (see fig. 9.8b).

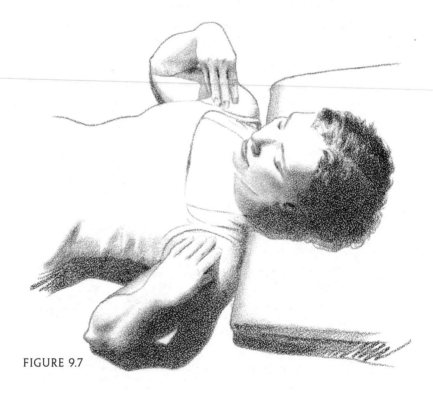

FIGURE 9.7

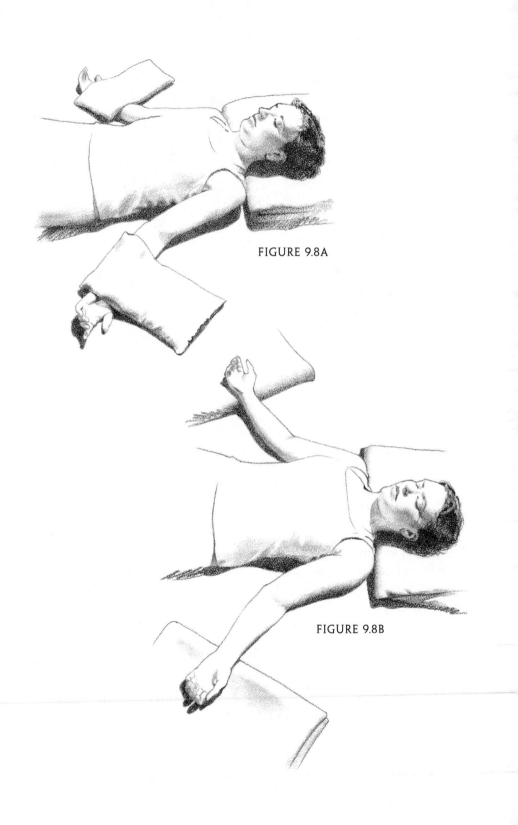

FIGURE 9.8A

FIGURE 9.8B

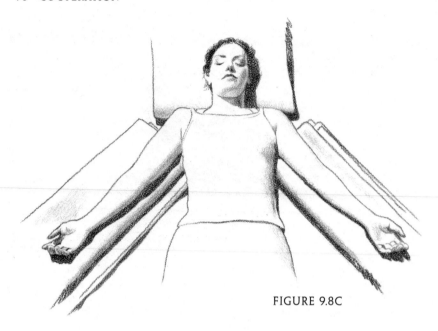

FIGURE 9.8C

- Fold two blankets widthwise three times, then lengthwise once. Angle them at forty-five degrees relative to your torso, then lay the arms and the backs of the hands on these supports (see fig. 9.8c).

Spend a minute or two with the arms resting on the floor, the heads of the humerus bones sinking deep into the scapulas. Next rest your index fingers on the manubrium, your pinkies on the xiphoid, and the middle and ring fingers on the body of the sternum. How much space is there between your sternum and your scapulas? Watch the fingertips rise and fall with the inhales and exhales. Then fan the entire bone away from its midline, push the manubrium up toward the head, the xiphoid down toward the navel. Remember that you're raising the top sternum, not the bottom. Most beginners, when asked to open the chest, will poke the bottom sternum and the lower front ribs forward. This actually sinks the upper chest and overarches the lower back.

Then spread your fingertips across the bottom borders of the clavicles, pinkies near the sternum, index fingers near the acromions. Spread the clavicles away from the sternum. How wide are you across the shoulder tips? The clavicles are often narrowed and glued to the two top ribs, which dimples the fronts of the shoulders where they join the torso. This pinches the breath in the upper chest.

Here's where you'll want to open the eyes of the heart, the areas just below the clavicles to either side of the sternum. First pull down on the top ribs just below the clavicles, as if you were pulling down on your lower eyelids. Then, as you continue to push your feet lightly against the floor and scrub the scapulas down the back, push the clavicles up, away from the top ribs, as if you were pushing up on your eyebrows. Watch the clavicles slide over the tops of the shoulders and feed into the scapulas. Imagine that the clavicles are lifting the front of the shoulder yoke away from the rib case. Breathe into the upper ribs.

Finally return your hands to the floor, palms up.

HOW IT HELPS

This is a very versatile exercise. First it teaches us the three significant actions of the scapulas, which are to: press into the back toward the sternum, widen across the back, and slide down the back toward the tail. Second, the exercise teaches us to root the arms in the mid-back (rather than the shoulder joints), and integrate their movements in the heart. Finally, it helps us to soften and create space in the upper chest (the eyes of the heart) which, as one aspirant wrote, "gives me more room for air."

Caution. Be sure not to squeeze the scapulas together to help widen the sternum and clavicles, especially when sitting. Also, don't push the lower front ribs and the xiphoid forward, out of the torso, to help lift the top of the sternum and clavicles. Remember to lift the top of the sternum and the manubrium, not the bottom at the xiphoid.

When sitting for pranayama, some students have a tendency to lift the shoulders during inhalation. Imagine that there's a weight hanging from each of the scapulas. Slide these bones down toward the tail on the inhalation.

Spine

The spine has thirty-three vertebrae. Each vertebra has a body and three bony projections, called processes, two to either side of the body and one behind, like a tail. The spine has five sections: the cervical, with seven vertebrae; the thoracic, with twelve vertebrae; the lumbar, with five vertebrae; the sacral, with five vertebrae (fused in adults); and the coccygeal with four (or sometimes five) vertebrae (also fused in adults) (see figs. 9.9a and b).

The spine also has four sides. It's not hard to imagine the right and left sides, but the back and front may need some explaining. We can easily see and touch the back spine. Take a look at your back torso in a mirror. That line of little bumps down the middle of your back from the top of your neck to the pelvis is the tips of the vertebral tails. Because we can see them so easily, they give the impression that the spine is just below the surface of the back, but this is misleading. Actually the bodies of the movable vertebrae, along with the fused bodies of the sacrum, are nestled deep inside the torso. So the front spine, which follows the front line of the vertebral bodies, is buried out of sight and out of reach.

Seen from the side, the spine has four curves: in the neck, rib case, lower back, and sacrum. Technically, then, the front spine follows a sinuous path from its base at the coccyx to its apex at the atlas, the aptly named first cervical vertebra. But for the purposes of this guide, and to make our practice easier, we'll think about the front spine as a straight line from the middle of the pelvic floor to the atlas.

PRACTICE

Cross your arms over your chest, as if you were hugging yourself, but don't grip the sides of the shoulders with your hands. Feel the shape of your torso, using the hands, arms, and floor as tactile aids. Imagine that it's a slightly flattened cylinder, wider across from side to side and narrower from front to back.

Look into the inner space of your torso. Imagine two sheets of glass, one that divides the torso in half from front to back, another that does the same from side to side. Can you find where these two sheets

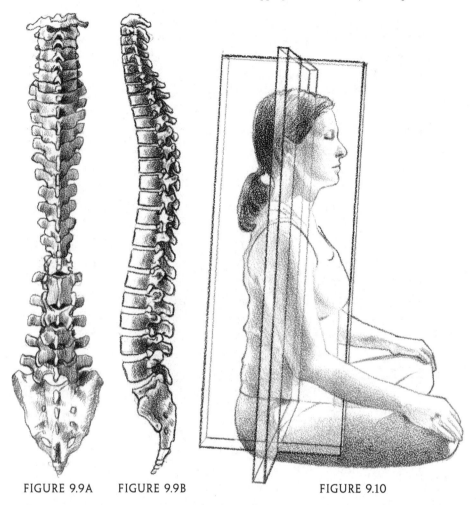

FIGURE 9.9A   FIGURE 9.9B   FIGURE 9.10

intersect? This is the line of your front spine, your midline, what I call
the heart axis. Extend this line in two directions, down through the bottom of your pelvis and up through the crown of your head (see fig. 9.10).

Now rock slowly from side to side. You can push your feet against
the floor to help get yourself going. First, feel just the back of your
torso and how it seesaws on the floor. Can you find the fulcrum of
this movement? It's right along the line of the back spine. Then shift
your attention to the front spine and watch how your torso-cylinder
rotates around its heart axis. Go back and forth for a few minutes,
watching first the seesaw rocking on the back spine, then the cylinder rolling around the front.

Gradually come to a stop with the weight of your torso balanced evenly on the back spine, half to the right and half to the left. Lay your arms out to your sides. Push your feet lightly against the floor. As the back spine scrubs down from the base of the skull to the coccyx, watch the front spine lift up from the coccyx to the base of the skull at the atlas. Always remember the spine mantra in everything you do: "Up-the-front, down-the-back."

HOW IT HELPS

The two circuits of the spine reflect our two greatest human urges, to ascend and transcend or climb above the material world and to descend or incarnate, to flesh ourselves out, in and with the world.

In the sitting position the down-the-back action anchors the spine through the lengthening tail into the center of the earth, stabilizing (sthira) our seat. Up-the-front lengthens our central channel, the heart axis, inducing a sensation of ease (sukha) and lightness, in the sense of both weightlessness and illumination. This length, in turn, frees the respiratory diaphragm.

Mr. Iyengar notes that it's the job of the spine to "keep the brain alert." This means that the spine isn't just a physical structure but a psychological one as well. The moment the front spine collapses, the brain collapses, too, and the intense awareness needed for pranayama and meditation vanishes.

The two spinal circuits serve as a kind of measuring stick against which we can gauge the moment-to-moment fluctuations of our skillfulness, not only in our yoga practice but in our everyday lives as well. The circuits support each other. To go only up-the-front is to pull away from the earth, to lose contact with our physical base; to go only down-the-back is to sink into the earth and lose contact with the self.

Caution. Be careful not to lengthen the front spine artificially by pushing the back spine into the body, which thrusts the lower front ribs forward, or widen the back spine by collapsing the top chest and narrowing the shoulders. Remember that the front and back of the torso should widen equally.

Neck and Head: Hyoid, Inion, Atlas

Just as there were several important landmarks on the pelvis, so are there on or in the neck and head.

The hyoid is one of the more interesting bones in the body. Hyoid actually means "shaped like the letter upsilon," the Greek U. It's a small, horseshoe-shaped bone at the crook of the neck, where the underside of the chin meets the front of the throat. The only bone in the body not jointed to another bone, the hyoid is the root of the tongue and an attachment for several neck muscles.

The inion is the little bump on the back of your skull just above the hollow in your neck. Did you reach for the back of your head as you read that last sentence? The next time you have the chance, ask a friend, "Do you know what that little bump on the back of your head is called?" See what happens.

In Greek myth the Titan Atlas supported the heavens on his shoulders. In our body the atlas supports the skull. You can't touch the atlas, but you can get a feel for it. Simply nod your head "yes, yes, yes" over and over, making only a very small rocking movement. On the bottom of your skull are two small bumps, called the occipital condyles. As you nod, these bumps are rocking back and forth inside two small indentations in the atlas. You can think of the occipital condyles as the sitting bones of your skull.

PRACTICE

Press your thumbs to the base of your skull. Spread your fingers across the sides of your head. Pull the skull away from the back of the neck. Then rest your head a few inches off the floor on a folded blanket or firm pillow to relax the neck and throat. Angle the underside of the chin perpendicular to the floor. The head, like the torso, should be balanced on its midplane. Check that the ears are equidistant from the tops of the shoulders, so the head isn't tilted and the sides of the neck are equally long, and the eyes are equidistant from the ceiling, so the head isn't turned to one side or the other.

Touch the tips of your index fingers to the crook of your neck, just

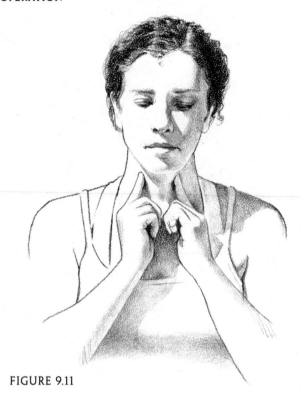

FIGURE 9.11

below and slightly in from the angle of the jawbone. Poke gently back and forth a few times to find the horns of the hyoid. If it eludes discovery for now, don't worry (see fig. 9.11).

Now press your thumbs on either side of the inion and splay the fingers across your temples. Lift your head an inch off the floor, pull the inion away from the nape, and slide the skin of the back skull toward the crown. The skin of the nape releases away from the base of the skull. Return your head to the floor.

Lightly press your fingertips on the horns of the hyoid and lift the bone diagonally into the skull. This simple action triggers a circuit that includes the entire head and spine. (see fig. 9.12). From the crook of the throat (1), the circuit passes across the atlas (2) to the inion (3). Here, at the back of the skull, the circuit divides: half flows up the back of the head to the crown (4) and ultimately down across the forehead (5), inner eyes, corners of the mouth, over the chin and back to the hyoid; the other half flows down the back spine to the tail (6).

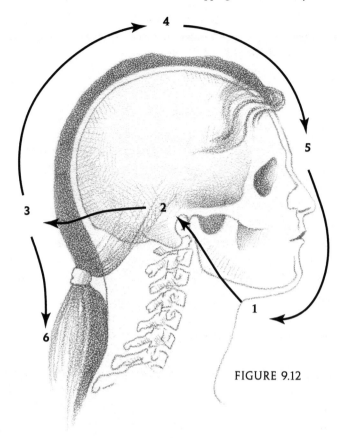

FIGURE 9.12

We'll come back to this circuit (in chapter 20) as a preparation for the Net-Bearer Lock (jalandhara-bandha).

HOW IT HELPS

The next time you're walking down the street or sitting in a restaurant, take a look at the people around you. Notice in particular the relationship of their heads to the rest of their bodies. Line up an ear hole with the seam along the shoulder line of a shirt or jacket, or just with the head of the upper arm bone. It's very common for our head to be well ahead of the rest of us as we go bustling through our normal busy day. Informally this head-shoulder imbalance is called forward head, and it leads to all kinds of problems, like chronic headaches and jaw joint pain.

The head should never be a side load on the spine. The actions here help to rebalance the head where it belongs, on the top of the spine. They also soften the throat and tongue and lengthen the back of the neck.

GOING FURTHER

Once you've adjusted yourself in Corpse and fidgeted and scratched as much as you need to, resolve to stay as still as possible for the duration of the practice. Remember that both balance and stillness are essential elements of Corpse.

Take a few minutes to experience the embrace of gravity and the quality of your contact with the floor. What's it like? Do you feel comfortably down to earth, or are there places that seem up in the air? How would you describe what you feel, or how would you map it out?

Then imagine that your body is filled with a thick fluid, like honey or motor oil. Sink this mass into the pull of gravity and let it settle down onto and spread across the floor, so that the front of your body grows light and spacious, and the back heavy and broad.

To come out of Corpse, bend your knees and roll with an exhale to the right side. Wait for a few breaths. Then lift yourself from the side, using the strength of your arms to push your torso away from the floor. Drag your head and brain up last. Perform Corpse at the end of each practice, whether asana or pranayama. Many years ago I was taught, as a rule of thumb, to do five minutes of Corpse for every thirty minutes of practice.

LAST WORD

It's not easy, as you probably discovered in the last chapter, letting go of the gross body in Corpse, at least not if you're just starting out on your practice. Though they're not recorded in any of the older guides, it's a well-established fact that there are what are called "Corpse gremlins" that do everything in their power—make your nose itch, induce uncontrollable coughing or sneezing fits, and just in general mess with your mind—to upset your relaxation. Don't despair. As your practice progresses, they gradually lose their hold over you and one day disappear.

Some students actually like to draw their body maps; others just write them out. Accept that your first few attempts will probably look something like world maps from early sixteenth-century Europe, with the shapes and sizes of the continents strangely distorted and large areas labeled "Terra Incognita" or "Here Be Dragons."

We'll get to some exercises in chapter 14 that will support the work you've just finished here.

CHAPTER 10

Quieting the Sense Organs in Corpse

The next level of the practice is becoming proficient in Turning the Senses inward in order to temporarily sever the link between your mind and senses, and external stimuli. . . . This enables you to separate and disentangle yourself from the conflicts and contradictions that are occurring in the mental field so that you can look down into the Lake of the Mind and become aware of thoughts and feelings that you are not normally aware of.

—Patanjali, *Psychology of Mystical Awakening:*
Patanjali Yoga-Sutras, translated by Swami Savitripriya

THERE'S ONE further element in the equation of a successful Corpse, the quieting of the five traditional sense organs—the skin (at the bridge of the nose), eyes, nose, tongue, and ears.

The yogis refer to the five sense organs collectively as the *jnana-indriya.* You may remember that *jnana* means "wisdom" or "knowledge." When we hear the word wisdom, we usually think of someone who's read a library full of books, and we certainly can say that this person is brimming with jnana. But when the yogis use this word, they're usually referring not to worldly wisdom but instead to spiritual insight or gnosis, a word that's often adopted to render jnana into English and that, if you look at its spelling carefully, you'll see is a distant relative.

The second part of the word refers to Indra, whose name means "Ruler," and whose place in the Vedic pantheon is much like that of Zeus among the ancient Greeks. The jnana-indriya, then, supply us with wisdom about both the world around us and the country of the Self and, when all is said and done, are pledged to the service of the divine.

According to the yogis, our sense organs, especially our eyes, aren't merely passive receptors of worldly information. Our surroundings don't simply pour into us like water into a cup; instead, the organs also play an active role in our perceptions of people and things, reaching out like the tentacles of an octopus to grab onto the objects of our attention.

Every perception we have of the world generates a corresponding fluctuation in consciousness. When I look at a chair, for example, a chair-shaped vritti is propagated in my citta—and there's the rub. Our very contact with the outside world through our sense organs is a major breeding ground of the dreaded vrittis, which keep us in thrall to our spiritual ignorance.

So the yogis, ever looking for ways to diminish their fluctuations, practice what's called sense-withdrawal (pratyahara), the fifth limb of Patanjali's eight-limb system (see chapter 2). In effect, they retract their senses and sever their engagement with the world, a technique that's often pictured as a tortoise pulling its limbs and head into its shell.

I know this may seem like extremely weird behavior. But given the operating premise of the classical system—that the fluctuations get in the way of authentic self-knowledge—it makes perfect sense. Pratyahara is a logical extension of asana and pranayama, the third and fourth limbs of classical yoga. All three practices are designed to deprive citta of any and all external stimuli, whether motor or perceptual. The yogi, like the tortoise, retires into a shell and simply refuses to be distracted by the world. She commits herself to attend only to the inner world of consciousness in a search for ultimate self-truth.

Through the practice of pratyahara, says Patanjali, the yogi attains "supreme obedience" (Yoga-Sutra 2.55) of the sense organs. Then, remarks Vyasa, "just as bees follow the course of the queen bee and rest when the latter rests, so when the mind stops the senses also stop their activities."[1] Sense-withdrawal attenuates the causes of our spiritual affliction by disrupting the normal flow of our consciousness. The practice continues the process, initiated with asana and pranayama, of deconstructing our surface self so that the authentic self can emerge.

We won't, of course, be attempting a full-blown version of sense-withdrawal here. That might be a bit much to ask of ourselves at this stage. Rather, I'll give you a few simple exercises for your five sense organs that will give you a feel for sense-withdrawal. All of the following exercises should first be performed and perfected in Corpse, then transferred to the sitting position when you reach that stage in your practice.

Skin (Tvac)

The yogis call the space at the bridge of the nose the interval between the eyebrows (bhru-madhya). It's a favored foundation (adhara), a place where they fix and so steady the eyes during meditation and pranayama. It's also the site of the sixth major energy center, the command wheel (ajna-chakra), and the third eye, or eye of wisdom (jnana-cakshus).

For the time being, we're only concerned with the physical space. Anatomists call it the glabella, which roughly translates as the "bald spot." The psychologist Paul Schilder, whose classic studies of the human body image are reported in *The Image and Appearance of the Human Body,* mentions that we localize our ego, our surface self, at the glabella.

You'll need the following props: a blanket or towel rolled up thickly enough to support the natural curve of your neck, a block, and a sandbag.

PRELIMINARY

Before you try this exercise, you might take a look at yourself in a mirror. What does the skin at your glabella look like? Is it soft and smooth, like a baby's skin, or is it creased and wrinkled from too much care and hard thinking? If I asked you which way the skin seems to be moving—inward toward the midline of the forehead or outward toward your temples—what would you say?

PRACTICE

Use your fingertips to gently rub and spread the skin of your glabella. Imagine that it's melting away from the midline of your forehead, over the temples and ears, and down onto the floor.

HOW IT HELPS

The muscle that covers the forehead (called the frontalis) tends to tighten up under stress. Over time, as the stress continues, the muscle becomes extremely tense. Softening the skin at the glabella quiets the brain and helps the body as a whole to relax.

GOING FURTHER

Here's a heavy-duty technique to soften the skin of the forehead. Support your neck on a rolled-up blanket. Stand your block on one side directly behind your head with its long axis parallel to your spine. With your fingertips, as you did earlier, gently spread the skin away from the midline of the forehead and release it toward your temples. Then lay the sandbag on the block with its long axis parallel to the block. Pull the sandbag a little farther down onto your forehead, scrubbing the skin toward the bridge of the nose (see fig.10.1). Stay for five minutes. Continue to watch, in your imagination, how the glabella softens and slides toward both the bridge of the nose and the temples.

For another glabella-releasing technique, we'll work with the Six-Openings Seal later in the chapter.

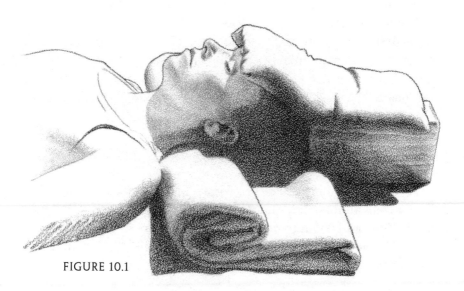

FIGURE 10.1

Eyes (Cakshus)

Most of us look out at the world through our eyes and assume that what we see is what we get. But to the yogis, our material world is just the thinnest veneer on the surface of existence. They are able to see, with the eye of wisdom, into the subtle heart, what Sri Aurobindo calls the Divine Being, of things and people. Though everyone has this yoga eye, it's opened only by concerted yogic practice or, as in the case of Arjuna in the Bhagavad-Gita, the grace of God.

The eyes are connected to the brain through the optic nerve. A wandering gaze, claim the yogis, disturbs the peace and quiet of the brain. And so they steady the eyes—just as they steady the body in asana—by directing their gaze (drishti) toward one of two points, the interval between the eyebrows (bhru-madhya) or the tip of the nose (nasa-agra).

PRACTICE

For this practice you'll need an eye bag or a folded towel. While it may be traditional to gaze with crossed and open or half-open eyes at the forehead or tip of the nose, it's not very easy to do. With your fingertips continue stroking downward from the bridge of your nose across the inner eyes and cheeks. Do this several times.

Then cover your eyes with an eye bag. Imagine that they're sinking heavily into their cup-shaped sockets. Even with the eyelids closed, the eyes may still move around, generating more fluctuations. Turn your eyes down and gaze into the inner space of your torso at your heart. The yogis call the heart the city of Brahma (brahma-pura). Inside this city is a lotus, in which is a secret place, often pictured as a cave or cavity (guha). Here, in the deepest recess of our being, dwells our authentic self, the atman, purusha, or puri-shaya, she who reposes (shaya) in the being as in a city (pura). The heart resident is said to be very small, smaller than a grain of rice, but at the same time greater than all the world. Look carefully. In this way you'll quiet the fluctuations and begin to develop your own wisdom eye.

Despite your best effort to keep the eyes turned down, they may return to their wandering ways after a while. Be persistent. After some practice you should be able to hold the eyes in a steady downward gaze.

HOW IT HELPS

Softening and then down-turning the eyes helps to quiet the skin of the forehead and the brain and, like pratyahara, draw awareness inward toward the self.

Caution. Some students report that turning the eyes downward hardens them. If this happens to you, then imagine that you're turning the eyes backward and gaze at a fixed spot on the inner lining of the back of your head. Make sure your eyes don't puff up in the inhale like two little balloons. Drop the eyeballs heavily to the back of the eye sockets and keep them there throughout your breathing session.

GOING FURTHER: SIX-OPENINGS SEAL (SHAN-MUKHI-MUDRA)

One traditional technique used to quiet the senses for pranayama and meditation is called the Six-Openings Seal (shan-mukhi-mudra). This seal is so-called because six openings of the head—the two ears, two eyes, and two nostrils—are sealed with the hands (to see a picture of the traditional technique, look in B. K. S. Iyengar's *Light on Yoga* under "Shanmukhi Mudra"). Usually it's performed in the sitting position, but we'll do the seal here while reclining. Too, we'll work with a modified technique. Instead of using our fingers for the seal, we'll substitute an elastic bandage, a prop developed by B. K. S. Iyengar, which will seal only the ears and eyes.

PRACTICE: MODIFIED SIX-OPENINGS SEAL

Here are two versions of this modified seal. The first is for aspirants working only with the skin of the forehead or those who for whatever reason can't or won't wrap their eyes. The second version is for the forehead and eyes.

Forehead Only

Roll the bandage into a tight roll. Hold the roll in front of you with the free end in your left hand and the roll itself in your right (reverse the instructions if you're left-handed). Press the free end against the back of your head, then unroll the roll across the right side of your head and across the top of your ear, your forehead, the left side of your head and the top of your ear, then back to the back of the head. Keep wrapping in this way until the entire roll is wrapped around your head. Tuck the free end of the roll under an edge of the wrap (see fig.10.2).

Forehead and Eyes

Finish one wrap, as instructed above. Then, for the next wrap, angle the roll up across your right eye after crossing the bottom of your ear, across the bridge of the nose, down across your left eye and the

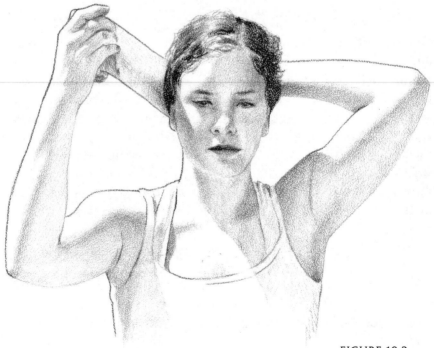

FIGURE 10.2

bottom of your ear to the back of the head again. Do this again for the third wrap and tuck the free end of the roll under an edge of the wrap (see fig.10.3).

Pull down just slightly on the wrap so that it scrubs the skin of your forehead toward the glabella. Release the eyes away from the wrap toward the back of the head.

HOW IT HELPS

Traditionally Six-Openings Seal is used to seal consciousness, to prevent it from leaking out into the world, and stimulate the subtle inner sound (nada), which serves as a seed for meditation. In this guide the seal is used to partially block outside sounds and light and soften the eyes and skin of the forehead. This helps quiet the brain and calm the fluctuations of consciousness. One aspirant wrote in her journal that "I feel secure and nurtured" when wrapping the head with the bandage.

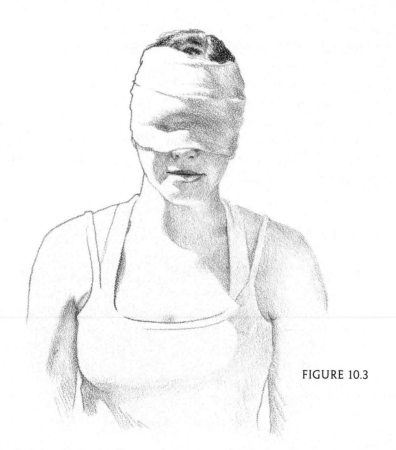

FIGURE 10.3

If you're suffering from a headache, try Six-Openings Seal. Wrap yourself in one of the two versions and lie in modified Corpse for fifteen to twenty minutes. With slow breathing (see chapter 12), imagine that your head is shrinking inside the wrap.

Caution. While you can wrap the forehead fairly tightly, wrap the eyes lightly. Remember to cross the wrap over the bridge of your nose, but don't wrap or in any way block your nostrils.

GOING FURTHER

B. K. S. Iyengar mentions that the brain is the hardest part of the body to adjust. Most people believe that the brain is, as he says, the subject—in other words, the source of consciousness. But as he continues, our brain and consciousness are everywhere, diffuse throughout our body, and the "head" brain is in fact an object of perception, just like a leg or an arm.

When using the Six-Openings Seal in Corpse, imagine that your brain is sinking onto the back of your head, growing smaller with each inhalation. Finally your brain is the size of a pea—or any other small object, if you object to the idea of a pea brain—surrounded by the vast inner space of your skull.

Channel your inhales away from the brain. Imagine that a tube leads away from each of your nostrils directly down into the torso, so that the breath and brain are kept away from each other. You can also sink and shrink your brain with the sandbag on your forehead, as described above in the "Skin" section.

Nose (Ghrana)

I don't suppose that many of us think about tension in our nose. But we can and do tense our noses, as strange as that might seem, and this does have an effect on the way we breathe. The little rounded bumps on the sides of your nose are called the wings (alae, singular ala). These wings should be soft and passive during both quiet breathing and pranayama.

PRACTICE

From the inner corners of your eyes, gently stroke with your index fingertips down along the sides and wings of the nose and continue along your upper lip to the corners of the mouth. Do this several times, each time releasing the wings downward. Be sure to keep the wings moving downward as you breathe, especially on the inhales.

HOW IT HELPS

Softening the wings of the nose helps the breath flow more easily into and out of the body. Remember that the breath is pumped into and out of the body by the diaphragm, with its roots deep in the lower back, not by the nose.

PLAYING AROUND: NOSTRILS

You've also probably never been asked, Where do the inhales and exhales touch on the inner linings of your nostrils? Most normal people don't think about this issue, but the yogis, who think about a lot of odd things, do. According to the yogis, the five traditional elements—earth, water, fire, air, and space—are found in various localized spots on the inner lining of the nostrils (see *Light on Pranayama* for one example of this). Experienced breathers can, by channeling their inhales and exhales over these different element-sites, affect the quality of their consciousness.

This requires, as you might assume, a fair amount of sensitivity, a little beyond what's expected of beginning breathers. But we can still begin to get a feel for this technique with a simple exercise. Through the years I've learned several ways to channel the breath over the linings of my nostrils.

One teacher had us divide each nostril into an inner portion, against the septum, and an outer portion, under the wing. On the inhale we were instructed to direct the breath over the lining of the inner nostril, on the exhale over the lining of the outer. The claim here is that these two channelings help to deepen the space of the inhale and smooth the texture of the exhale.

Another teacher once drew us a picture of the shape of the nostril and noted that in outline it has much the same shape as a lung. He asked us then, in order to fully fill and empty our lungs, to breathe by touching the entire lining of each nostril with each inhale and exhale.

Notice how these techniques, and ones of your own devising, affect the qualities of your breath and chart these effects in your journal. Can you, for example, truly increase the space of your inhale by moving the breath over the sides of the septum?

Tongue (Jihva)

The tongue is involved in one of the strangest practices of Hatha-Yoga. It's called the Space-Walking Seal (khecari-mudra). A number of these seals are described in the old Hatha guides, with names like the Tank Seal, the Frog Seal, and the Crow Seal. We'll look at a couple of locks (bandha), the seals' close relatives, in chapter 20.

The tongue is attached to the floor of the mouth with a band of tissue called the frenum, the Latin word for "bridle." The yogis—or some of them, anyway—cut through this membrane over a period of months, while at the same time they pull the tongue out of their mouth with a pair of tweezers to gradually lengthen it. This is called milking the tongue, and in this context the tongue is compared to a cow (go). According to Gheranda, if you do this long enough—and I'm certainly not recommending it here—it's possible to eventually touch the space between your eyebrows with the tip of your tongue.

I know this sounds like an impressive enough feat, but wait, this isn't the actual seal yet. What these yogis do next is to turn this elongated tongue back in their throat, slip it behind the soft palate and into the skull cavity (kapala-kuhara). Since the tongue is equated with a cow, this technique is aptly called eating the cow meat (go-mamsa-bhakshana).

Once the tongue is inside the skull, the yogis use it to stimulate the base of the brain, which drips a miraculous fluid called immortal (amrita). Khecari-mudra, says Gheranda, "prevents fainting, hunger, thirst and fatigue. There comes neither disease, nor old age, nor death. The body becomes radiant."[2] There's more, but I think you get the picture.

I'm afraid that what we'll be doing for the tongue in this guide is much tamer.

PRACTICE

Your tongue is rooted deep in the throat at the hyoid bone (see chapter 9). Open your mouth wide and stretch your lips. Stretch your tongue out from its root with a long exhaled HA sound, as if you were huffing your breath on a mirror to clean it. Try to touch the tip of your tongue to your forehead . . . just kidding. Feel your tongue's length and width. Curl the tip of the tongue down toward your chin.

Then pull your tongue back into your mouth and release your lips. Be sure not to press the lips together. Keep them relaxed and slightly parted. Imagine your mouth then is expanding, as if you were yawning. Soften the root of the tongue and rest its tip behind the lower teeth. Imagine that it's spreading across the floor of the mouth, and from its tip, release along the sides of the muscle to its root.

HOW IT HELPS

Softening the tongue helps relax the throat.

GOING FURTHER

You don't have to cut your frenum and milk your tongue to experience the Space-Walking Seal. Exhale, curl your tongue back in your mouth, and touch the tip as far back in the cavity as you can. Take an inhale. Notice that with the tongue rolled back toward the soft palate, the inhale penetrates more deeply into the lower belly. Repeat a few time and then release the tongue again onto the floor of the mouth.

Ears (Shrotra)

Just as there's a subtle world of matter beyond the scope of our everyday eyes, so also there's a subtle world of sound beyond the range of our everyday ears. This divine symphony of subtle sound (nada) is accessible only to our yoga ear, which like all other yoga organs, is only developed after years of dedicated practice. But we can start, even at this early stage of our practice, to contact this special ear and hear faint echoes of the music of the gods.

Physically the ear has three parts: the outer ear, which is called the auricle (little ear) or the pinna (feather); the middle ear, also called the tympanum (drum), which has the three ossicles (little bones) that connect the eardrum to the inner ear; and the inner ear, with the spiral-shaped cochlea (snail).

I like to pretend there's a channel from each of my inner ears that feeds into my yoga ear, which I locate in the center of my skull, just at the top of the spine. When I tune in to the sibilance of my breathing, whether in formal practice or just sitting reading a book, I always try to focus the sound deep inside my head.

PRACTICE

Let's start with your physical ears. Imagine that the auricles are like two little pinwheels on the sides of your skull, joined by an axle passing through the two ear holes. Touch a fingertip to each tragus, that little projection just in front of the ear hole. Gently stroke down to the lobes, up the back of the auricle, around the top, and down to the tragus again. Repeat several times. Then watch your ear pinwheels turning from back to front.

Now shift your attention to your inner ears. What do they feel like? This probably won't be a question you can answer right away. Give it some time. Eventually you want the inner ears to feel very soft and deep. Imagine a channel from each of the inner ears to the center of your head, just between the ear holes. Draw your inner ears along these channels, toward the center of your head, into your yoga ear. Practice listening to the sound of your breath from here. Perhaps, after a while, you'll be able to pick up other sounds, too.

Svatmarama maintains that after about two weeks of listening for the subtle sounds—he may be a bit overly optimistic with this time frame—the fluctuations of consciousness are quieted and you feel great pleasure. What will you hear? He lists the sound of the ocean, next clouds, drums, a gong and horn, tinkling bells, a flute, and the humming of bees.

HOW IT HELPS

The wide-open eyes monitor and adjust the position and alignment of the body during asana practice. In pranayama the eyes are closed, so the ears step forward to play the role of monitor and adjuster, closely attending to the everyday sound the breath makes as it enters and leaves the body.

GOING FURTHER

Occasionally you might have some difficulty releasing your inner ears. There's also a channel from your inner ears down to your groins, so that thickness in one is usually reflected in thickness in the other. If one or both of your inner ears is reluctant to release, try to soften the same-side groin or groins. If the groin or groins, too, are unyielding, weigh them down with sandbags. Be sure to use an equal amount of weight on both thighs.

LAST WORD

This concludes our minicourse on Corpse. I won't pretend that it's any easier to work with the senses than it is to work with the rest of the gross body. It's a challenge to consciously turn them down while in the waking state, and then when you finally do, you risk drifting off into the twilight zone or falling asleep and losing touch with your Witness. But as with everything else you've done so far and will do later on, time, patience, and regular practice are the keys to success.

CHAPTER 11

Qualities of the Breath
Time, Texture, Space, and Rest

> The phases of breathing are exhalation, inhalation, and suspension. Observing them in space, time, and number, one is able to render breathing more harmonious in duration and subtlety.
>
> —Patanjali, *The Essence of Yoga:*
> *Reflections on the Yoga-Sutras of Patanjali,*
> translated by Bernard Bouanchaud

ARE YOU READY to begin pranayama? I know I've disappointed you with this question twice already, but here, at last, is our first look at the *what is* of the everyday breath. And you may notice that, as you take this look, although you're not purposely doing anything, your breath will subtly change. In the lions, elephants, and tigers approach, we always let happen before we help happen and make happen.

We'll look at four qualities of the everyday breath in particular: time, texture, space, and rest. I recommend, though, that you continue with these quality exercises only if your Witness is well established, at least in Corpse (that is, if you can lie relatively quietly in Corpse for at least fifteen minutes and enjoy it), and you have a reasonably accurate map of your body's surface features and its inner space.

So if your Witness and Corpse are still unsteady, or if your body map still has large areas marked "Terra Incognita," it's probably best to stop right here. Feel free to read the material in this chapter and beyond, but put off moving on until you have achieved the desired level of control.

Spend at least a week or two exploring the following qualities and return to them now and again as your practice develops. Set aside at least fifteen minutes each day for practice, preferably after your asana practice, though just about any time is OK as long as you don't rush. Remember that your practice will go much smoother later if you take the time in the early stage to make sure you have a good axle hole.

There are several ways you can organize your practice sessions. For individual sessions you can focus on one quality only for the entire session or work with two, three, or all four qualities in each session. Then, over the longer term, you can stay with the focus quality for several sessions—say, a week's worth—or cycle through each of the four qualities over every four-day period. You can also pay more attention to any of the qualities that are especially difficult for you. For example, spend one day on time, two on texture, and then three on space.

HOW IT HELPS

When we focus on something that interests us, our breath tends to slow down, smooth out, and even stop altogether. Watching the qualities of the breath has the same effect on the breath itself. As the breath slows, smooths, and stops or comes to rest, the fluctuations of citta do the same, loosening the grip of avidya and revealing more and more of the answer to the question Who am I? One aspirant reported that he actually forgot to breathe, because the rest was so blissful.

Caution. Take the time to look at the qualities thoroughly. Some students are in a hurry to begin "real" pranayama. They go right to the later stages without first laying a quality foundation, and their practice often suffers. First find out what is. This is also part of the answer to the question Who am I?

Don't despair if the qualities elude you at the start of your practice. Have patience and practice regularly, even if results are slim. Be careful not to struggle with the breath and try to force it into unbreathed layers or sections of layers.

While these exercises seem harmless enough, students do report problems. One common problem is with the slowed pace of the breath, which makes some students impatient and irritable. Whenever you feel these emotions, or any similar emotions, in your practice, stop immediately. Go back to everyday breathing in Corpse until you're relatively calm and end your practice for the day. Be sure, during the rest exercises, not to hold your breath, especially with muscular effort. That comes later, after much more training. For now just expand the natural rest for two or three more counts.

Four Qualities of the Breath

We'll look at the four qualities of the breath in the modified Corpse position. Be sure to do the following practices in the order in which they're listed—that is, time, texture and space, and rest. Simple observation of the qualities will by itself transform your breathing rhythm without any real effort on your part. Witness your time, and you'll find that it naturally begins to slow down. This is the key to the entire practice: when the time slows, you'll find the texture of the breath smoothing out, the space filling, and the rests lengthening. For these practices you'll need two blankets and whatever other props you want for Bent-Knee Corpse. You might also want one or two sandbags.

PRELIMINARY

Roll each blanket into a thin roll. Lie in Bent-Knee Corpse with whatever props you like. Put one roll under your lower back and one under your neck. The rolls should be thick enough to comfortably support the natural curves of your lumbar and cervical spines but not so thick that they increase the curves (see fig. 11.1).

Time

Time is the length or, as Vyasa says, "calculation of the moments" of the inhales and exhales (and retentions, which we'll include in chapter 20). According to Gheranda, we breathe on average 21,600 times a day, which is about 15 times a minute. Each breath, then, lasts four seconds. But take this traditional figure with a pinch of salt. Actually I read somewhere that men take a fifth fewer breaths than this number each day, while women take a third more.

The yogis have some interesting ways to time their pranayama breaths. For example, Vyasa mentions the moment (kshana), which is a technical term in classical yoga. Vacaspati Mishra, in his ninth-century commentary on Vyasa titled the "Clarity of Truth" (Tattva-Vaisharadi), reckons a moment as "one-quarter of the time required for the act of winking." A quarter of a wink! Try that only with expert supervision. Vacaspati also mentions a unit called a measure (matra), which is computed "by snapping the thumb and forefinger after having three times rubbed one's own knee-pan with the hand."[1]

In everyday breathing, time varies throughout the day, as our breath speeds up and slows down or stops altogether, depending on what we're doing and how we're feeling. In pranayama the first way we control (ayama) the breath is to slow it down. Later, when the unmeasured slow breath is established, we regulate first the relative lengths of the inhales and exhales (we'll get to ratio pranayama in chapter 17) and then the retentions (kumbhaka, in chapter 20).

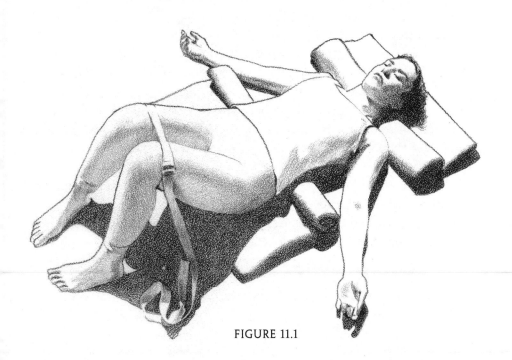

FIGURE 11.1

PRACTICE

As I said earlier, time is easy to figure out. During your inhale simply count one-OM, two-OM, three-OM, and so on, until the breath is complete (we won't do any winking or finger snapping in this guide). Count the same during the exhale, starting again with one-OM. Continue counting each inhale and each exhale for about a minute. Most people find that their exhale is slightly longer, by a count or two, than the inhale.

As you count, you may notice that something happens to your breathing. When we concentrate on our own breathing, its time tends to slow down. This slowing is, as I've already noted, the first thing we do to control (ayama) the breath in pranayama. Make sure that for now you don't try to slow down purposely; just let it happen. We'll do some deliberate slowing and talk about the implications of slowing in the next chapter.

Texture and Space

For convenience we'll combine the work with texture and space, but you can work with them separately.

In common usage texture refers to the feel or appearance of a surface or to the essential character or scheme of something. Of course, your breath itself isn't like the smooth or rough surface of an object, and so you can't run your hand over it and feel it. But you can feel, with or without your hands, the movement of the breath or, more precisely, the movement of the torso as the breath enters and leaves the lungs.

How do you find the texture of the breath, then? I'm sure you're aware of the movements of your breath, at least occasionally, maybe while lying in bed at night or in asana class. Unless you're very aware, though, all you experience are the gross movements—the big picture, so to speak. But just as your everyday consciousness-stream fluctuates as it flows, you'll notice, if you take a closer look at the details of your everyday breath, that it does something similar. Like our duhkha chariot, it bumps along the road, speeding up and slowing down and periodically even coming to a complete halt.

Since citta and breath or prana are, as we already know, intimately related, their vrittis are simply manifestations of the same disquiet provoked by avidya. According to Svatmarama, "When prana moves, chitta moves. When prana is without movement, chitta is without movement. By this (steadiness of prana) the yogi attains steadiness and should thus restrain the vayu (air)."[2]

So the second way we control the breath in pranayama is to smooth its texture as much as possible. Texture consists of both movement of the breath, from the beginning of the inhale or exhale to its conclusion, and balance of the breath, between the right and left halves of the torso; the front and back halves of the torso; and the lower, middle, and upper thirds of the torso.

Space or place (desha) traditionally has several meanings. It can refer to a place outside the body, which the yogis usually localize twelve fingers' or three fists' breadth from the tip of the nose, where the flow of the everyday exhale comes to an end. Here the space is called the external end-of-the-twelfth (bahya-dvadasha-anta). (There are two other external points, at the crown of the head and twelve fingers' breadth above the crown, which won't concern us here.) There's also a space inside the body, usually but not always localized in the heart wheel (hrdaya-cakra), called the internal end-of-the-twelfth (antar-dvadasha-anta). Finally, space can refer to the entire space inside the torso or the body as a whole. In this chapter we'll focus on the inner space of the torso, which we've already experienced somewhat from our mapping expedition (in chapter 9).

In everyday breathing we're mostly aware, when we're aware at all, of the space in the front torso—in the belly for some people, the chest for others. We tend to breathe in front because we're most conscious of this side of ourselves, which we see and touch easily and often. Our back torso, which we can't see and touch as easily, is riddled with avidya and so out of our everyday awareness and largely unbreathed.

The third way we control our breath in pranayama is to fill and empty the entire space of our torso, to use our breathing capacity to the fullest. I've emphasized fill and empty here because, obviously, we don't physically breathe air into our entire torso, but only the lungs. But the image we use, and after some practice the feeling we get, is that we're also breathing into and out of—and filling and emptying—the abdominal cavity.

Many students report that space is the most perplexing of the four qualities. It can't be measured like time, touched like texture, or witnessed like rest. To be successful with space, you need liberal portions of imagination and patience.

PRELIMINARY

We'll divide our torso into three cylindrical sections, like a three-layer cake. These layers are:

1. The lower belly, from the base of the pelvis at the perineum to a line circling the torso through the navel.

2. The upper belly, from the navel line to a line circling the torso through the base of the sternum; this section includes the lowest pairs of ribs.

3. The rib case, from the sternum line to a line circling the torso just above the clavicles.

PRACTICE

Lay your hands in turn on each of the layers. For the lower belly rest your hands to either side of and below the navel. On the upper belly, the pinkies should be just above the navel line, the index fingers just below the sternum line. For the third layer, slide your fingertips to the front upper ribs, just above the line of the nipples and below the clavicles.

For the first few minutes of each exercise, just witness the hands rise and fall with the inhales and exhales. Then, for each layer, ask yourself these general questions about the texture of your breath:

- Do the hands move at all when resting on the layer? Using the floor as a tactile aid, can you feel any breathing movement in the back half of the layer? Slide your hands to the sides of the layer. Any movement here?

- Now focus solely on the inhale. Again, any movement in the front, back, or sides? If there is movement anywhere, what's it like? Is it smooth from start to finish? Or do your hands rise and fall erratically, in fits and starts?

- Now, still focused on the inhale, divide your attention between your two hands. Watch them move. Any difference in the way they rise? Some students report, for example, that their right hand moves faster than their left, or the right moves faster for the first part of the inhale, then the left catches up. What about you? (For a variation of this exercise, see appendix 2, "Breathing with a Friend.")

- How would you describe yourself as an inhaler? How do you react emotionally to conscious inhalation?

Then shift your focus to the exhale and repeat these instructions and answer the same questions. Next shift your awareness from the surface movements of the container to its inner space. What, if anything, do you see (or imagine you see) or feel (or imagine you feel)?

Once you've worked through all three layers, lay your arms and hands to your sides on the floor. For a few minutes, inhale and exhale up and down through the layers. Smoothly transition the breath up from the lowest belly to the heart and clavicles on the inhale and back down in the reverse order on the exhale.

GOING FURTHER: LOWER BELLY

One commonly cited obstacle in the lower belly is a feeling of darkness in the bottom half. While the breath penetrates into the top half of their lower belly just below the navel line, students report that the bottom half just above the groins seems cut off. One student wrote in her journal, "My breath gets a little below the navel and just stops dead, like it's hitting a wall." A likely physical cause of this is tightness in the groins and pelvic floor (which we'll work to open in chapter 14). For now, if you meet this obstacle, get two sandbags and lay them on your groins, parallel to the crease, so that they form a V with the apex at the pubis. The weight should help to soften the groins and descend the breath.

GOING FURTHER: UPPER BELLY

Students regularly detect a hard spot just below or at the lower tip of their sternum, at the attachment of the front diaphragm. On the inhale this spot seems to sink into the torso as the rest of the upper belly rises, squeezing the movement of the breath. There also seems to be a strong emotional charge associated with this spot, which is mostly expressed in the journals as sadness and longing. For now, if you meet this obstacle, get your elastic bandage or a small wash-cloth and roll it up into a tight roll. As you lie in Bent-Knee Corpse, position the little roll under your back, just opposite the hard spot, with its long axis parallel to your spine. Then rest your fingertips on the spot and imagine that it's like a little belly. On each inhale soften and puff it. Be sure not to force the breath into the hard spot if it insists on resisting and certainly don't push forcefully against it with your fingers.

GOING FURTHER: RIB CASE AND CLAVICLES

Students often remark that the upper half of their rib case feels stuck. As one student wrote, "There's no room for the breath." Lots of people, including many yoga students, are very flat and narrow across the upper chest. That's because their clavicles have sunk in toward the sternum and down on the top two pairs of ribs and are, as one of my teachers used to say, glued in place. (We'll do some stretches for this area in chapter 14.) For the time being, if glued clavicles are a problem, try the following floating ribs exercise.

Floating Ribs Exercise

Since the floating ribs are attached only to the spine and not to the sternum, they rotate in their joints easily during breathing. This very ease of movement can be used to coach the movement of the other ribs, especially the top two pairs, which are short and thick and, as you may have discovered, not easily breathed.

Direct your Witness to the lumbar roll. The floating ribs are just above this roll. For a few minutes, breathe into your lower back. Watch the movement of the floating ribs, using the roll as a tactile aid. On the inhale they expand outward, much like a pair of kitchen tongs being opened, and on the exhale they close. See if you can feel (or imagine you feel) the free and easy movement of the floating ribs.

Next rest your fingertips on your upper chest, just below the clavicles. Breathe—or at least try to breathe—into your fingertips. What is your breathing movement like in these two pairs? Probably not much like the way it was with the floating brethren. Now see whether you can re-create the movement of the floaters in the ribs just below the clavicles. Pretend that the tails of the top pairs of ribs where they join the sternum are, like the floaters, unattached. As you breathe into your fingertips, watch them swing freely up and down.

Now shift your awareness from the surface movements of the container at the ribs to its inner space. What, if anything, do you see (or imagine you see) or feel (or imagine you feel)?

Rest (Vishrama)

When most of us think about breathing at all, we usually think about its two active phases, the inhales and exhales. But as I've mentioned, there are also two resting phases in the four-phase cycle, the inner rest after the inhale and the outer rest after the exhale. Rest is a hiatus that separates the inhales and the exhales, the brief time-outs that the diaphragm takes with every breathing cycle as it goes about its business of keeping us alive and breathing.

If inhale and exhale is our breath's way of doing something, rest is its way of doing nothing. Rest provides us with an opportunity to understand the what is of breathing more fully. I imagine that the active phases are like the letters in a sentence or the notes in a song, while the rests are the spaces between the letters or notes. We couldn't read the letters or hear the notes without the spaces, and space by itself would have no shape or meaning.

PRACTICE

As Patanjali suggests, the movement of breath sustains or breathes life into the fluctuations of our objective and subjective realities. As soon as that movement ends in rest—especially in the deep rest of kevala-kumbhaka—our reality also rests.

Breathe normally for a few minutes, witnessing time, texture, and space. To begin the exercise, for the first few minutes, watch the rest at the end of the inhale. Then, again for a few minutes, shift your Witness to the rest that follows the exhale.

You may notice that, just as the other three qualities are transformed by witnessing, so, too, is rest. After a while you may detect that the rests between the inhales and exhales are expanding, without any conscious effort on your part. Many students report that these expanded rests are exceedingly satisfying. For example, one student wrote in her journal, "I got so comfortable in the outer rest that I didn't want to take the next in-breath. I just wanted to stay there, suspended, calm."

GOING FURTHER

Rest is a kind of precursor to kevala-kumbhaka, which is nothing more than a deliberately planned and extended rest designed to foster the restriction (nirodha) of the citta-vrittis in classical yoga or restrain the prana in the pot and intensify its transformative power in Hatha-Yoga. One aspirant discovered that "God is in the space between the breaths."

Ask yourself these questions about rest: What feelings arise during my rests? Some students, like the one I quoted earlier, relish their rests, while others are understandably disturbed by the moment of deathlike stoppage of the breath.

What happens, if anything, to the fluctuations of my citta during the rest? Can you understand why the classical yogis put such a heavy emphasis on fixing (stambha) their breathing in their quest for the restriction of the vrittis?

PLAYING AROUND: FOUR QUALITIES

Play around with the four qualities as you go about your daily business. Do this in different kinds of situations—at work, in a store or post office, standing in one of those interminable lines, or in your car, which I consider to be absolutely the best laboratory for yogic experimentation and application. Forget about Himalayan caves and forest monasteries; anybody can be steady and comfortable in one of those places.

Notice when the breath is disturbed, when it speeds up, when it becomes rough or shallow, or when it stops altogether. What does this breathing say regarding your feelings about or reactions to the situation or person at hand? Who is the breather now? Try to flip the breathing on its head—consciously slow the time, smooth the texture, open its space. What happens when you do this, if you can?

One of my teachers once compared the breath and consciousness to the two prongs of a tuning fork. Tap one of the prongs, he said, and the other begins to vibrate. Then squeeze one prong with your fingers, damping its vibration, and its mate will also stop vibrating. Is this your experience of the relationship between breath and consciousness? Can you really affect the latter by altering the former, not only in the controlled setting of your practice room but also in the unpredictable, and sometimes unmanageable, everyday world?

LAST WORD

Write about your experiences with these four qualities in your journal. You'll probably find that your ideas about them change from day to day at first, but eventually you should be able to get a pretty clear profile of what they're like and how they reveal your breathing identity.

Remember the importance of listening in pranayama. Don't only witness the inhales and exhales but also listen to the sound the breath makes as it passes through your nostrils. (We'll work further with this sound and amplify it into a mantra or hymn in chapter 17.) The sound has two important functions in pranayama: it absorbs and inwardly focuses both our fluctuating consciousness and the usually outgoing senses, and helps us monitor the texture of the breath through slight variations in pitch.

CHAPTER 12

Unusual Breathing

If, when I am in a hurry, something suddenly arrests my attention and arouses my interest, I immediately slow down, just as I would slow down in a car if I passed through interesting scenery. And this mental act of slowing-down has the immediate effect of revealing fine shades of meaning that I had previously been in too much of a hurry to notice.

—Colin Wilson, *G. I. Gurdjieff: The War against Sleep*

I HOPE BY NOW you have a well-drawn map of your body and everyday breath. Without it you stand a good chance of taking wrong turns, stumbling over obstacles, or missing points of interest as you venture through the country of the Self.

With this map in hand, so to speak, you should be ready to begin to purposely control (ayama) your breath for the first time. While the initial stage of the lions, elephants, and tigers approach is a necessary prelude to pranayama and the resolution of our avidya, witnessing and letting happen aren't sufficient by themselves as a means of liberation. We still have to use the map and apply what we've learned, and venture out bravely into the country of the Self. In other words, as the yogis tell us repeatedly, our success also requires that we make things happen.

The four exercises in this chapter, though, are really a kind of transition between let happen and make happen. While there is effort involved in the exercises, the level of that effort is fairly low. So rather than make happen in the exercises that follow, you'll cooperate with the breath and help happen, to refine and expand your understanding of what is and further reveal and realize what could be.

As you may have discovered, it can be difficult to step back from our breath and discern its qualities, even with the help of the

Witness. We get so habituated to our breathing identity that our awareness of it gradually shrinks and almost disappears. What do we do then? We need an exercise that's out of the ordinary or unusual, that introduces something new into our everyday breathing behavior and so shoots it back up into consciousness. The four unusual-breathing exercises in this chapter change, either subtly or by exaggeration, the everyday qualities of the breath and so help to highlight our breathing identity. I call them stop-and-wait breathing, slow breathing, zigzag breathing, and spot breathing.

Stop-and-wait breathing is a continuation of the rest exercise in the previous chapter and a further preparation for kumbhaka, or retention. The exercise involves both extension of the natural rest and inhibition of all doing. The word inhibition has a bad reputation nowadays, but I'm not talking about the kind of inhibition that suppresses otherwise healthy behaviors, impulses, thoughts, desires . . . and breathing. Remember our charioteer from chapter 1? His job, in effect, was to inhibit the boisterous behavior of the horses and get them harnessed (yoga) to the chariot. The charioteer became, over time, the prototype of the yogi, who is diligently at work restricting (nirodha) the similarly wild fluctuations of citta. Our inhibition here is similar to classical nirodha, which will rein in unnecessary or harmful behaviors, impulses, thoughts, or desires.

I'll never forget the first words out of the teacher's mouth in my first ever pranayama class: "I can't teach you how to breathe." Great, I thought (because I was too timid to say it out loud), where do I get a refund? But he was making a key point that I didn't understand at the time: no one can teach you how to breathe, because you already know how. The yogis would say that breathing is an inherent capacity or potential of the universe that manifests in almost all living creatures.

Each of us is initiated into the breathers' circle at birth, spontaneously in tune with, though not conscious of, our authentic breath. Breathing obstacles, whether physical or mental, are usually, though not always, self-created. In the lions, elephants, and tigers approach, we don't begin by practicing some new breathing exercise but instead clarify and map the what is, warts and all, of the surface breather. Then, with this knowledge firmly in hand, we inhibit whatever's unneeded or harmful about our breathing behavior and get out of the way of our own authentic breath. We can't learn how to breathe, but we can learn how to stop not breathing, to rein in our surface breather and wait for our authentic breath to breathe us.

Slow breathing, as the name suggests, is a deliberate slowing of the everyday time of your breath. The time exercise in chapter 11 may have shown you that when you closely witness your breathing—whether in terms of its time, texture, or space—it tends to slow down spontaneously. But you can also reverse the exercise. By intentionally slowing the time quality of your breath, you can intensify your Witness and so reveal finer shades of meaning in your breath.

Zigzag breathing needs some explaining. You may have discovered, in the texture exercise, one or more irregularities—bumps or jerks or halts—in your everyday breath. Relatively speaking, though, everyday texture is smooth from the beginning of the breath until its end. Zigzag breathing isn't—on purpose. Each complete breath is interrupted at regular intervals by a short reverse breath: the inhale with exhales, the exhale with inhales.

This exercise is based on, and so is also a preparation for, Against-the-Grain (viloma) pranayama (which we'll work on in chapter 19). As the name suggests, Against-the-Grain runs counter to our normal way of breathing: the inhales and exhales are measured out in steps, interrupted at regular intervals by measured rests. In zigzag breathing, as I've mentioned, the rests during inhale are replaced by short exhales, and the pauses during exhale are replaced by short inhales.

Spot breathing is a continuation and an intensification of the space exercise. In spot breathing we'll direct our Witness and the breath to specific spots in the torso.

All of the breathing exercises in this chapter should first be performed and perfected in Corpse. Later they can be repeated, if you feel it's necessary or beneficial for your practice, in the sitting position.

Gather whatever props you want for Bent-Knee Corpse. Optionally you might have a sandbag and a couple of blankets handy.

PRELIMINARY

Lie in Bent-Knee Corpse for all of these exercises. Breathe normally for a few minutes before you start, witnessing time, texture, space, and the inner and outer rests. Always begin the exercise, as you'll begin formal pranayama, with an inhale. Remember that each practice session has four stages: warm-up, main, review, and relaxation.

HOW IT HELPS

In general, unusual breathing breaks the habitual rhythm of our everyday breath and captures our interest. This strengthens our Witness so that we can expand and refine our breathing clarity.

Most of us try too hard to breathe—we have to learn to make less of an effort. So unusual breathing teaches us how to let the breath just happen, to trust in our authentic breather. Finally, it suggests new breathing possibilities and begins the formal training of the breath and readies it for the more demanding practices of pranayama.

Caution. Even though the level of control in the following exercises is very low, some students don't like control very much at all. Be aware of and write about your own reactions to these exercises. If you feel put off by control, it may be that for some time to come—months or even years—your pranayama practice will consist mostly of letting happen under the watchful eye of the Witness.

Other students have trouble with slow breathing. Slow inhale tends to increase the space of the breath, and not all new breathers are ready and willing to become more spacious. They report that taking in, or at least trying to take in, more breath than usual is met with enormous physical and emotional resistance and causes headaches, irritability, or anxiety. Slow exhale, on the other hand, intensifies letting go or surrender. While many students can take in easily enough, surrender, giving (whether of the breath or the identification with the surface self) is almost impossible and again is resisted—even resented—mightily.

What are your reactions to taking and giving? Remember that the physical breath has powerful emotional and spiritual associations. Be sure not to ignore or avoid any taking or giving issues that arise. Go slowly with these exercises and the pranayamas that follow. Take time to connect with your Witness before each session. That will automatically slow your breath. Don't push beyond what you perceive to be comfortable breathing limits. And resolve to spend at least a few weeks—or if necessary, a few months—on these exercises before proceeding to the pranayamas.

Stop-and-Wait Breathing

In the rest exercise, you witnessed and let happen only the rest itself. To get ready for the stop-and-wait exercise, first extend the time of your rests. The count should be less than or equal to (but not longer than) your lower time count, whether it's inhale or exhale. In other words, if your time count is, for example, four for the inhale and five for the exhale, your rest count would be four. Then attend especially closely to the end of each rest, right before the inhale or exhale commences. We'll work on the outer and inner stop-and-waits separately.

PRACTICE: OUTER STOP-AND-WAIT

The assumption in this guide is that we all do something unneeded or harmful that inhibits our authentic breath. This doing something usually belongs to our breathing avidya. Before we can go on to the higher stages of pranayama, we have to learn how to inhibit this inhibition and free our authentic breath.

To continue with this example, once you've established your four-count rest at the end of the exhale, watch yourself very carefully in the moment just prior to the inhale. Students report a wide variety of doings at this crucial juncture—some pretty obvious, others much subtler. The physical doings are ordinarily fairly easy to contact, though don't be lulled into thinking that they can't be subtle as well. Most commonly they involve gripping or tensing one or more of the sense organs, the throat, areas of the torso (especially the shoulders, belly and groins), or the limbs.

There are also psychological doings, which might be harder to catch. Even in the reclining position, balanced nicely on our midline, with our head and eyes bandaged up, our groins weighted down with heavy bags, we still tend to make a psychological effort to take a breath.

As usual, don't do anything for the first few minutes; just witness these doings. Make a mental note of what you find and watch how the doing affects each inhale. Then, when you feel confident that you have some understanding of what's happening, stop or inhibit what you're doing and simply wait for the next inhale to breathe you. Carry on for a few minutes more, perhaps shifting back and forth between doing and stop-and-wait.

PRACTICE: INNER STOP-AND-WAIT

Inner stop-and-wait is just the reverse of outer. Focus your Witness on the moment just before the exhale and again, when you're ready, stop doing and wait for the breath to breathe you.

It goes without saying, though I'll say it anyway, that it may take you some time to track down all of your breathing avidya, which is deeply ingrained in consciousness. You might stick with physical avidya for the first week or so of the exercise.

HOW IT HELPS

The stop-and-wait exercises help us chop habitual breathing avidya off at the root. It's well known that it's easier to inhibit the unneeded or harmful inhibition before it builds up a head of steam.

Caution. Don't struggle bug-eyed to prolong your rest. Avoid escalating any already existing muscular gripping or tension in the name of inhibition. Remember that the ultimate stop-and-wait, kevala-kumbhaka, is natural and nondeliberate.

Work a good while with the two stop-and-wait breaths before you move on to the next breaths.

Slow Breathing

Slow breathing is a key preparation for all the later and more challenging pranayamas. You may have already discovered that if you simply witness your everyday breathing, the breath tends to spontaneously slow itself down. Slow breathing is like running a video in slow motion: it lets you see things that may have escaped your notice when the action was viewed at normal speed.

PRACTICE

This exercise is divided into two parts, which work first on the inhale and then on the exhale. For both parts take a minute or two to establish your everyday time. Let's say, as an example, that your inhale count is three and your exhale count is four.

PRACTICE: INHALE

Add one count and inhale for four counts. Breathe for a few minutes, counting and watching texture and space. If the four count is comfortable, then add another count, so that you inhale for five counts. Continue on in this fashion, adding one count at a time, then inhaling to that count for a few minutes with each addition, until you reach what you feel is the edge of your comfort limit. Then back off by one count. Witness the inhale for a few minutes more with this last count, then return to everyday breathing.

Remember here that you're working on the inhale. Exhale as you always do, although you may notice that as the time of your inhale increases, so does that of your exhale.

PRACTICE: EXHALE

Everyday exhale is largely an elastic recoil of the energy generated by the contraction of the diaphragm and other respiratory muscles during inhale. In this exercise and in formal pranayama, we'll actively control the release of the inhale-generated energy during exhale.

Add one count and exhale for five counts. Breathe for a few minutes, counting and watching texture and space. If the five count is comfortable, then add another count, so that you exhale for six counts. Continue on in this fashion, adding one count at a time, then exhaling to that count for a few minutes with each addition, until you reach what you feel is the edge of your comfort limit. Then back off by one count. Witness the exhale for a few minutes more with this last count, then return to everyday breathing.

Remember again that you're working on the exhale. Inhale as you always do, although you may notice that as the time of your exhale increases, so does that of your inhale.

HOW IT HELPS

Slow breathing streamlines the breath and automatically smooths its texture. Slow exhale in particular increases our opportunity to extract more oxygen, and so energy, from each breath; purifies the lungs of stale air and toxins; and helps us relax physically and mentally. It gives us a chance to take a breather and reduce our normally breathless pace.

GOING FURTHER: THREE SLOW-BREATHING EXERCISES

Here are three exercises that support slow breathing: belly weight, roots and rim of the diaphragm, and eyes of the heart.

PRACTICE: BELLY WEIGHT

In chapter 11 we used our fingertips to monitor the rise and fall of our belly during everyday breathing. There we were concerned strictly with the texture and space of the breath. Here a sandbag (or other weight) replaces the fingertips and is used as a tactile aid to purposely modulate the movement of the breath. For props use some kind of light weight, either a sandbag or a book (maybe even this book, if you don't have a bag), as a tactile aid.

Lay the bag across your lower abdomen with its long axis perpendicular to the line of your spine, below your navel, above your pubis. Again work with your inhales and exhales. During the inhale exercise, watch the bag rise, slowly and steadily like an elevator ascending from the ground floor to the roof. During the exhale exercise, first lift the bag with an everyday inhale and then, as you exhale, lower the bag, again like the elevator, slowly and steadily from the roof to the ground floor (see fig. 12.1).

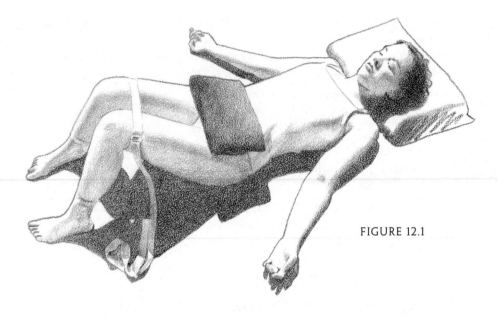

FIGURE 12.1

Caution. Be careful whenever you breathe with a weight on your belly, even if it's only everyday breathing. Some students report that the weight is distracting or restrictive and that, rather than illuminating their breathing behavior, it darkens it even more.

PRACTICE: ROOTS AND RIM OF THE DIAPHRAGM

We won't go into the diaphragm in too much detail. There are five physical diaphragms in the body and, as some yogis claim, at least that many subtle diaphragms. The one we're talking about here is technically called the thoracic or respiratory diaphragm. If you want to know more about our primary breathing muscle, refer to the books in the "Recommended Reading" section of this guide. For our purposes here's what's important.

Look at the accompanying illustration of the diaphragm. You'll immediately notice its unique appearance and central location in the torso. Notice first that the right half of the muscle is slightly higher than the left, to accommodate the large bulk of the liver. It's been imaginatively described in various ways: as a double dome, an umbrella, the lopsided cap of a mushroom, and a jellyfish. These images, remember, describe the muscle at the end of an exhale, since on the inhale the muscle flattens out (see fig. 12.2).

Diaphragm literally means "fence through," an allusion to its position in the middle of the torso, between the abdomen below and the chest or thorax above. In function we can compare the diaphragm to a piston inside a cylinder, the torso. As we inhale, the diaphragm contracts and flattens about an inch or so, pushes down against and balloons the abdomen, and expands the interior volume of the chest both vertically and horizontally. This lowers the inner pressure of the thorax below that of the outside air, creating what's called a pressure gradient, and air flows in. As we exhale, the diaphragm releases and, with the help of the contracting abdominal muscles, pushes up into the thorax, changing the pressure again, and air flows out. The more the diaphragm can freely move, the more the lungs will expand and the more oxygen we can assimilate on each breath.

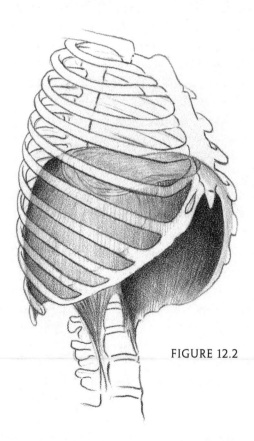

FIGURE 12.2

It's a bit misleading to characterize the diaphragm as a fence, because it doesn't really divide the torso into two distinct territories, like my neighbor's property and mine. With its up-and-down motion, it's more accurate to say that the muscle rhythmically integrates the spaces and vital organs, both subtle and gross, situated above and below. When the diaphragm is restricted or frozen—whether through injury, poor posture, or emotional stress—this integration is hindered, and we feel anxious or depressed or tired and disconnected from ourselves and others.

If you look at the diaphragm from the side, you'll see that it crosses the torso diagonally from higher in the front at the xiphoid to lower in the back at the lumbar. There are two long, stringlike muscles that extend down from the back rim of the diaphragm and attach it to the lower spine. These are the crura (singular crus), a word that means "legs" or "shanks," which I like to think of as the roots of the diaphragm. Mabel Todd, author of the classic study of human body structure and movement *The Thinking Body*, says of the crura that "because of their shape and position, the action of the crura is more easily comprehended than that of any of the other muscle fibers of the diaphragm. It is their contraction that is most definitely involved in the pulling downward of the top of the dome of the diaphragm."[1]

For this practice you'll need a rolled-up blanket, thick enough to support the natural curve of your lower back. Lie on the rolled blanket so that your lower back is firmly supported. The roots of your diaphragm are right above this roll on either side of your spine. Soften and widen the muscles of your lower back. Now recall the illustration of the diaphragm and its pair of roots growing down along the lumbar spine. Exhale slowly and, to initiate the next inhale, imagine that you're pulling down on the roots and that they, in turn, pull down on the diaphragm. As the dome of the diaphragm flattens on this inhale, watch the breath flow upward from the lower back to the top of the shoulders. At the end of the inhale, gradually slacken the pull on the roots and exhale down along the back spine to the lower back again. Continue in this way for a few minutes.

Next spread your hands on your lower front ribs. The rim of the diaphragm attaches all around the bottom of the rib case, slightly higher in front at the lower end of the sternum, lower in back at the floating ribs. Though it's shaped much like a kidney bean when seen from above, you'll have to pretend that the rim is circular.

Again inhale from the roots. Imagine now that the circular rim of the diaphragm is expanding evenly outward from its exact center in the middle of the torso. Keep the center very soft as you actively increase the diameter of the rim, until the inhale is complete. Then on the exhale slowly shrink the circle in toward its center. Continue for a few minutes.

PRACTICE: EYES OF THE HEART

The eyes of the heart, remember, are just below the clavicles to either side of the sternum. They open wide to receive the inhalation and on the exhale stay open to prevent the air from rushing too quickly out of your lungs.

Rest your fingers on the eyes of the heart. Pull gently down on the upper two pairs of ribs and imagine that they're sliding away from the clavicles. Then push up on the clavicles and imagine that they're sliding up and over the tops of your shoulders. Pretend that the eyes of the heart are opening wide and gazing up at the ceiling in delight and wonder.

Next breathe into these eyes. You can keep your fingers on the eyes for tactile aid. On the inhale open the eyes even further. On the exhale, even as the breath flows out of the lungs, keep them open as completely as you can for as long as you can. The wide-open eyes of the heart prevent the chest from collapsing too quickly on the exhale. We'll come back to these eyes in later chapters.

Spot Breathing

Recall the three layers of the torso:

1. The lower abdomen, from the base of the pelvis at the perineum to a line circling the torso through the navel.

2. The upper abdomen, from the navel line to a line circling the torso through the base of the sternum; this section includes the lowest pairs of ribs.

3. The rib case, from the sternum line to a line circling the torso just above the clavicles.

Divide each of the three in half, either down the middle into right and left halves, so that you have three right and three left halves, or down the middle into front and back halves, so that you have three front and three back halves.

PRACTICE

Start spot breathing with any one of the six halves. Let's start, for example, with the right half of the lower abdomen. For a few minutes imagine that your inhales are channeled directly, and only, into that half layer. Touch the half layer with your right fingertips if you need tactile aid. Next, for a few minutes more, shift your Witness and your breath, and your left fingertips if needed, to the lower left abdomen. Then return to everyday breathing and witness the lower abdomen.

What would you say about yourself as a right-lower-abdomen breather and a left-lower-abdomen breather? How do the breaths in the two half layers compare?

Move to the upper abdomen and then the rib case and repeat these instructions. You could also reverse the order of exploration and start with the rib case and work down.

Another way to work with the side-to-side halves is to do the right halves first, from bottom to top or top to bottom. Imagine that your breath is moving only through your right nostril. Once you've climbed either up or down through all three right-side half layers, repeat the same process with the left-side half layers, imagining that your breath is moving only through the left nostril. Finally, return to everyday breathing.

You can also practice with the front and back halves of the torso. You might want blanket rolls under your lower back and neck for tactile aids. Start with the back lower abdomen and, just as you did for the side-to-side exercises, work your way up through the three layers a half layer at a time. Channel the breath over the back of the throat when you breathe into the back halves and over the front of the throat for the front halves.

PLAYING AROUND

Anytime you purposely change the everyday rhythm of your breathing, there's an element of play involved. I suppose you could say that pranayama itself is breathing play, though indeed a highly stylized form of play. The unusual-breathing exercises in this chapter are meant to be playful, too, though so far you've played entirely by my rules.

In the spirit of play, then, I'd like to give you an opportunity to express your own breathing playfulness. Let's take spot breathing and open it up a little more so that you can experiment and improvise on your own, according to your inner promptings.

Start by quartering—in your imagination, of course—each of the three layers of the torso, so there are right-front and left-front and right-back and left-back quarters. This makes twelve quarters in the torso in all, which together represent your field of play, like a chessboard.

Lie on your back as you did before and look at the twelve quarters. As the breathing spirit moves you, hop your breath around in these quarters. For example, you could breathe into

- One quarter of a single layer
- Two quarters of a single layer at the same time, like the right-front and left-back quarters
- Two quarters of different layers at the same time, like the right-front lower abdomen and the left-front upper abdomen

The possibilities for breathing play, as you can see, are myriad. What kinds of interesting patterns can you create with your breathing in these quarters?

Zigzag Breathing

This exercise is divided into two parts, which work first on the inhale and then on the exhale. Before you begin zigzag breathing, perform slow breathing with awareness of texture and space to your most comfortable count for a couple of minutes. Let's say, for example, that your slow inhale count is six, and your slow exhale count is eight.

PRACTICE: INHALE

Inhale for two counts. Then zigzag the breath by exhaling for one count. Again inhale for two counts, then again exhale for one count. Continue on in this way until you've inhaled for a total of six counts and, during the inhale, exhaled for a total of three counts. Work with these counts for a few minutes. Then see if you can add another layer of counts, so that you inhale for a total of eight counts and, during the inhale, exhale for a total of four counts. Continue to add counts (in this example two for the inhale, one for the exhale) until you reach a comfortable limit.

After each zigzag inhale, exhale to your slow exhale count. Then take two to three everyday breaths before the next zigzag. As your practice progresses, you can reduce the number of these everyday breaths until, if it's possible for you, they're eliminated altogether.

PRACTICE: EXHALE

Exhale for two counts. Then zigzag the breath by inhaling for one count. Again exhale for two counts, then again inhale for one count. Continue on in this way until you've exhaled for a total of eight counts and, during the exhale, inhaled for a total of four counts. Work with these counts for a few minutes. Then see if you can add another layer of counts, so that you exhale for a total of ten counts and, during the exhale, inhale for a total of five counts. Continue to add counts (in this example two for the exhale, one for the inhale) until you reach a comfortable limit.

Before each zigzag exhale, inhale to your slow inhale count. Then take two to three everyday breaths before the next zigzag. As your practice progresses, you can reduce the number of these everyday breaths until, if it's possible for you, they're eliminated altogether.

GOING FURTHER

Some students find that counting the time of their breaths is a distraction, that they can't really witness the breath if they're occupied with counting. I also like to do an exercise I call release zigzag breathing, which doesn't require counting. Let's take, for this example, the zigzag inhale.

First perform slow breathing for a few minutes. Notice, as each inhale progresses, any feelings of pressure building in the torso and groins, the throat, and head. Then begin the exercise but don't count. Instead, as soon as you feel any pressure in the torso, throat, or head, stop, exhale slightly until the pressure is released or at least lessened, then continue with the inhale. Inhale again until you feel the pressure build and again stop, exhale slightly until the pressure is released or lessened, then continue with the inhale. Proceed in this fashion until the inhale is complete.

Exhale slowly and smoothly. Then take two to three everyday breaths before the next zigzag. As your practice progresses, you can reduce the number of these everyday breaths until, if it's possible for you, they're eliminated altogether.

Zigzag exhales are just the reverse of zigzag inhales.

LAST WORD

Here we are at the end of the second stage of our journey. We've got our traveling companion, at least the rudiments of a map of the terrain ahead, and some basic, if still evolving, ideas regarding the identity of the breather. You might, in fact, want to take a breather here and spend some time clearing up any lingering questions and conundrums. But if you feel comfortable and relatively confident you're on the right track, by all means move on to Part Three. We'll be working with what might be thought of as the "platform" of breathing practice.

Comprehension

CHAPTER 13

Reclining Supports

So lying for us will be an activity, just as standing is. And as in all our activities, we will aim equally at inner openness for our own life processes and at sensitive contact with the environment.

—Charles W. Brooks, *Sensory Awareness:*
The Rediscovery of Experiencing

Three Reclining Supports

One of the most radical of Mr. Iyengar's innovations in the teaching of pranayama is the change in the aspirant's position in the early stages of his practice. Most modern guides to pranayama of which I'm aware follow tradition and instruct the aspirant to assume a sitting position in an appropriate asana. But in the lions, elephants, and tigers approach, beginning breathers are schooled to lie on their backs— usually, though not always, supported by a folded blanket or bolster. What are the reasons for reclining at the start of the journey?

If you've ever tried to sit steadily and comfortably, as Patanjali requires for pranayama, for just fifteen or twenty minutes, you probably quickly determined it was difficult if not impossible. Without proper training most of us would be decidedly unsteady and uncomfortable—slumping, fidgeting, scratching, feet numb, aching in the knees and back—all of which would further contribute to the already nearly overwhelming fluctuations of our citta. Our main concern wouldn't be the body or breath. Instead, we'd be peeking at our watch and waiting for the duhkha at hand to end.

It's much easier for us to be steady and comfortable, and so focus on our body and breath, lying supine. We get the feeling of being securely held by the floor and the embrace of gravity, which relaxes habitual muscular tensions and quiets our brain, and opens us up to new ways of being and doing.

I should note, however, that not all teachers are enthusiastic about reclining for pranayama. They point out that when you lie down, as if to go to sleep, and when you breathe slowly, as if you were asleep, many students tend to . . . go to sleep. This is certainly a problem for some students. One possible solution is just to get more sleep . . . at night. Another is to open your eyes and take a few deep breaths at regular intervals.

There are various ways to support the torso and head in the reclining position. In this chapter I'll describe three supports, which I call the wide support, the narrow support, and the step support.

Which of the three is just right for you? It's probably best to start off your practice with the wide support and stick with it until you're comfortable with your breath. Then you can move to the narrow support. The step support is useful on those days when your breathing feels stuck and you need a little extra kick to open the chest. Along with the supports, you can use any props you found useful for Corpse—for example, eye bag or elastic bandage, sandbags for the groins.

PRELIMINARY

Recall (from chapter 4) that a folded blanket has sharp edges and dull edges. When using one or more folded blankets as a reclining support, always lie so that the sharp edge (or edges) faces toward your back, not away from you. In all three of the reclining positions, be sure that your arms and legs form equal angles with your midline, which is defined by your spine. For example, both arms should make forty-five-degree angles with the midline. Also be sure that the midline of your head—a line drawn across your face from the middle of the chin, along the nose between the eyes, and splitting your forehead—is in line with the midline of your torso. Almost every beginning student has his head screwed on somewhat crooked.

PRACTICE: WIDE SUPPORT

For this practice you'll need a rectangular bolster, if you have one, or if not, two blankets. If you don't have a rectangular bolster on which to lie, you can make a wide support with two blankets. Fold one open blanket widthwise three times, then lengthwise once. You now have a bolster that measures about ten inches by twenty-six inches. Fold a second blanket the same way and stack the two blankets with the sharp edges slightly staggered so the bottom edge is an inch or two in front of the top edge. If you like, you can fold a third blanket four times widthwise as a support for your neck and head or use a small, firm pillow (see fig. 13.1)

HOW IT HELPS

The wide support provides a comfortably broad platform for the back torso, which stabilizes and helps balance the reclining position. It's also a great chest opener. In fact, you can lie on the wide support anytime you feel the need to stretch your heart and breathe more spaciously.

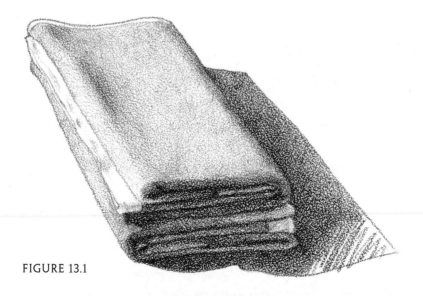

FIGURE 13.1

PRACTICE: NARROW SUPPORT

In this practice you'll only need a blanket for the narrow support. Fold your open blanket widthwise twice. You now have a rectangle that measures about twenty-five inches by forty inches. Lay it on the floor and look at the two long edges: one is sharp and the other soft. Kneel at the sharp edge, pick it up, and fold it away from you lengthwise, but don't fold the blanket in half: the bottom section should be about six inches wide, the top section about twenty inches. Fold the top section lengthwise back toward you, matching this new sharp edge to the first soft edge beneath. You now have two stacked or pleated sections, each six inches wide, and a third longer section of a little more than a foot. Fold this section lengthwise in half and lay the original sharp edge parallel to the original soft edge. Take a look at your blanket now from one end: it's folded neatly like an accordion and measures about six inches wide and forty inches long.

Finally, fold the top section in half, drawing that long sharp edge back toward you again, so that the new top section is about three inches wide. Pick this whole section up by sliding your fingers under that last fold and move it over the middle of the six-inch-wide base below. From an end view now, your blanket looks like a triangle, wide at the base and narrow at the apex (see fig.13.2).

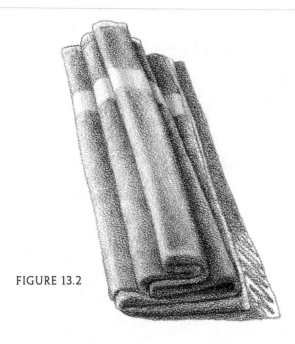

FIGURE 13.2

To support your head, either curl the head end of the support under the rest of the blanket to create a rounded lift for your neck or lay a second folded blanket across the narrow support under your neck and head (see fig. 13.3).

You can lie on the wide and narrow supports generally in one of two ways. To open the belly to the breath, sit against but not on the sharp edge of the support. Lie down so that your entire back torso and head are supported. You'll find that the belly and chest are at the same level.

Alternatively, to focus the breath in your chest, lie down so that the sharp edge of the support touches your back torso at a point opposite the lower tip of your sternum or against your floating ribs. The lower spine is unsupported, and the belly is slightly lower than the chest.

HOW IT HELPS

The ten-inch width of the wide support, while it encourages the chest to open, also presses against the back ribs and tends to restrict their movement during breathing. The narrow support is not as expansive, but since it fits nicely into the channel of the spine, it allows the back ribs to move more freely during breathing.

Caution. Since the narrow support is narrow, it's less stable than the wide support. Be sure that when you lie on this support, you carefully balance the weight of your torso so that you're not tilted to one side or the other. Imagine that the two sides of your torso are like the two pans of an old-fashioned scale. Rock from side to side when you first lie down, and slowly adjust the two sides of the torso

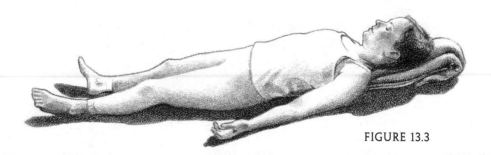

FIGURE 13.3

until they're equidistant from the floor and you're resting evenly on your midline, the spine.

Some students with chronic back pain find that the narrow support exacerbates their problem. If your back aches on this support, first bend your knees over a round bolster. If this doesn't help, then move off the support slightly, so that the firm edge is just below your sternum. But if the problem persists, move to the wide or step support (discussed below). Be sure to see an experienced teacher for some help with your back.

PRACTICE: STEP SUPPORT

For this support you'll need three blankets and a block. Fold one open blanket widthwise three times. Then fold it lengthwise in thirds: fold one-third of the length over once, then twice. The blanket will measure about nine inches wide by two feet long. Repeat with a second blanket. Fold blanket three widthwise five times.

Lay one of the two blankets on the floor. Place the block against the soft edge, with the long axis of the block parallel to the edge of the blanket. Stack the second blanket on the first, slightly staggered, so that the soft end sits on the block. Stack the third blanket on the second, on the block end, to complete the step support (see fig.13.4a).

Sit against the sharp edge of the bottom blanket and lie back. The middle blanket should support your scapulas, and the top blanket, your neck and head. Adjust the position of the top two blankets as needed (see fig.13.4b).

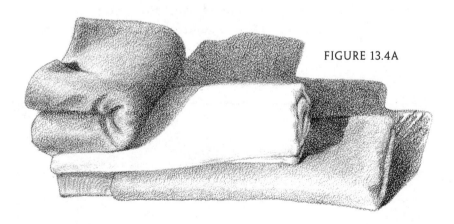

FIGURE 13.4A

Once your back is supported on any of the three supports, you can lay your legs straight on the floor, with the heels slightly apart, as you would for traditional Corpse. But you can also bend your knees and cross your shins one in front of the other in a cross-legged position. Then support your knees on thickly folded blankets or blocks. This position helps open the groins and lower abdomen. Or you can support the backs of the knees on a round bolster, with the outer heels on the floor. This position helps release the groins.

HOW IT HELPS

The step support, because of its width, is similar to the wide support. It's especially useful, as I've mentioned, for students who are (or temporarily feel) tighter in the chest and/or belly. Quite a few students find the step support to be the most relaxing of the three.

Caution. Be sure that the top blanket, the one supporting your head, isn't folded too thickly. That will tend to lift your head into a sharp angle relative to your neck, push your chin down onto your chest, and harden your neck and throat.

Transition from Reclining to Chair Seat

How long should you practice pranayama in a reclining position before you begin sitting in the Chair Seat? (See chapter 15.) That

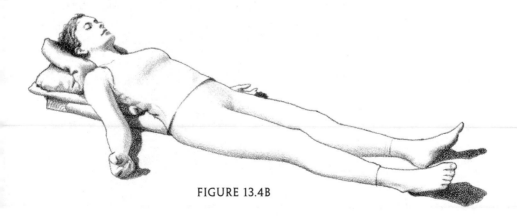

FIGURE 13.4B

depends on where you start from, your commitment to practice, and your karmic inheritance. There are two questions to ask: Do I have a strong asana practice? And do I have a strong reclining practice? In other words, am I preparing myself for the rigors of sitting, and can I breathe comfortably with Conqueror and Against-the-Grain, the two foundation breaths (see chapters 18 and 19), for fifteen to twenty minutes? You can probably expect to recline for at least the first four months of practice. Even after you've begun to sit and breathe, it's always a good idea to return to the floor periodically to check up on your breath.

If your asana and reclining practices aren't that strong, delay practicing in Chair Seat or any sitting position until you can confidently answer yes to the above questions. Be aware that the transition from reclining to sitting goes smoothly for some students but not for others. Even though you can answer yes to the above questions, there's still no assurance that you're ripe for Chair Seat. Don't despair if you run into obstacles. In the lions, elephants, and tigers approach, there's never any hurry.

LAST WORD

The three supports discussed in this chapter aren't the only ones possible. For example, you could also lie on the narrow support so that it's perpendicular to your spine instead of parallel, touching your back just a little bit below the lower tips of the scapulas. As you get more experience with the reclining position and the three supports, be sure to experiment with different supports of your own devising. Over the years I've tried cardboard rolls, various combinations of blocks, upside-down folding chairs, broomsticks, and other things I'm too embarrassed to mention. Remember that no idea is too exotic, though not every idea will work.

CHAPTER 14

Posture
Asana

There are eighty-four hundreds of thousands of Asanas described by Shiva . . . as many in number as there are numbers of living creatures in this universe.

—Gheranda, "How Many Asanas Are There?"
Gheranda-Samhita, translated by
Rai Bahadur Srisa Chandra Vasu

FORTUNATELY FOR US, Gheranda deems only 32 of the total 840,000 postures "useful for mankind." Modern guides usually describe anywhere from a few dozen postures to a couple of hundred, as in Mr. Iyengar's classic guide, *Light on Yoga*. Though it's likely that common sitting positions, such as Lotus posture (padmasana) and Perfect posture (siddhasana), are at least several thousand years old, nobody knows exactly when asanas first appeared. Some scholars speculate that the asanas originated in the yogis' spontaneous reactions to the current of divine energy streaming through their bodies in samadhi. Over the centuries this originally rhythmic, extemporaneous dance crystallized into the more or less static positions we have today.

Asana

Asana literally means "seat" or "sitting." Originally the asana was the yogi's meditation seat or platform, set up in a "clean place, neither too high nor yet too low, bestrewn with cloth or hide or grass."[1] Over time the word became associated with the physical position or posture itself assumed by the yogi, which is how we loosely define asana today.

In the classical system, asana is essentially a seat for pranayama and meditation. In his bare-bones outline of the classical system,

Patanjali devotes only three sutras to asana, expecting the guru to flesh out the details of the work: "The posture [should be] steady and comfortable. [It is accompanied] by the relaxation of tension and the coinciding with the infinite [consciousness-space]. Thence [results] unassailability by the pairs-of-opposites."[2]

The two classical criteria for a successful asana, as you can see, are that it be steady and comfortable (sthira-sukha). Each posture is a skillful balancing act between making happen and letting happen. This recalls the two great wings of classical yoga, exertion (abhyasa, which has the same root verb as asana) and surrender or dispassion (vairagya). When these two elements are in harmony in asana, the yogi relaxes or loosens (sithila) all physical and psychological tension; consequently the normally perceived boundaries of the body map dissolve, and consciousness expands to coincide (samapatti) with the consciousness that pervades all space, what Patanjali calls the infinite or endless (ananta). Then the yogi is free of the tug-of-war of conflicting pairs of opposites (dvandva), such as heat and cold, and can sit tranquilly for hours of pranayama and meditation.

Hatha-Yoga developed and elaborated the practice of asana beyond simple sitting postures. The yogi-architects of this practice believed that our body is a gift bestowed on us as a vehicle for self-liberation and that our first duty is to keep it healthy and preserve it for as long as possible. They emphasized health and longevity for two reasons: to buy themselves enough time to realize the arduous but priceless goal of their efforts, liberation, and to continue their existence indefinitely after reaching their goal and enjoy living liberation (jivan-mukti).

So the few seats of classical yoga burgeoned into hundreds of asanas, including many of the postures with which we're familiar today. Gheranda says that the asanas:

- Purify the body and destroy disease and death, which deliver us from the distractions and limitations of poor health and establish a hospitable physical environment for our training.

- Increase our digestive heat, the fire in our belly, which helps to assimilate whatever food we eat, whether physical or spiritual, more fully.

• Calm and energize the body-mind.

There's another reason for practicing asana, according to Hatha-Yoga. Remember that, as a means of liberation, the Hatha yogis shake and then awaken the mysterious sleeping serpent, kundalini. But unless our body is first prepared to receive this enormous charge of energy, it will crumble like "an unbaked earthen pot thrown in water."[3] So asana—along with pranayama and the seals (mudra)— "bakes" the body-mind, as the yogis say. It fosters physical and mental flexibility and firmness (dridhata), which release energy bound in both the physical and subtle bodies, and tune and condition the body to accept, process, and skillfully channel the increased energy of kundalini.

The Four Stages

We can apply the four stages, as we have in other contexts, to our work with asana. In stage 1 we witness and map the shape and structure of the physical body, the springboard of the practice of Hatha-Yoga. Asana is an unusual position that, like unusual breathing, introduces a novel element into our habitual ways of doing— of sitting, standing, and moving—and so clarifies these habits in our awareness. This also reverses the wandering (vyutthana, swerving from the right course) of citta and turns it toward the self. All yoga practice is like this: it keeps us immersed in and delighted by the process of transformation, which we recognize is accomplished both through our own efforts and through our acquiescence to a greater power. We feel more alive and so excited about the prospect of traveling beyond what we already know.

During stage 2 we work (cooperate) with the body to intensify and expand our range of familiar movements and add detail or color to our known world, and learn how we can do more with what we already know. At stage 3 we venture out courageously beyond the horizons of the known and take in hand (comprehend) the unknown, and explore the possibilities of a more spacious way of doing. Finally, in stage 4 we use asana to gradually penetrate into and integrate successively subtler levels of our incarnation, until all are in agreement with (and complete in) the self.

Keep these four stages in mind as you work with the postures. If you're still at stage 1, practice the postures as they're described, with no alterations, unless dictated by any special circumstances, until you understand their structure and intended effects. Then feel free to experiment and improvise.

HOW IT HELPS

Asanas are tools for self-investigation, self-transformation, and self-liberation. They also help us uncover and work with some of the physical and psychological obstacles, such as tension in the torso, imbalances in breathing between the two sides of the torso, and irregular or choppy and unfocused breathing.

Caution. As a general rule of thumb, stay alert for pain in the neck, lower back, and inner knees. If the correction I suggest doesn't seem to alleviate the problem, stop. Consult with an experienced teacher before you continue with that exercise.

Nine Asanas

We'll focus on nine asanas in this guide. They were chosen because they're accessible and fairly easy to do without the supervision of a teacher. Remember, though, that it's still tricky to learn from a book without a teacher watching and adjusting and that, while these postures are useful preparations for your breathing practice, they're not meant as substitutes for a regular, well-rounded asana practice.

These nine asanas help us to contact, stimulate, and realize (that is, make real) important areas of the breathing body. They'll stretch the front and inner thighs and groins, hips, abdomen, and the muscles between the ribs (intercostals); center the femur heads in the hip sockets; and reinforce the energy currents of the pelvis and shoulder yoke. At the same time, they're relatively passive positions that will open without tiring the body and help draw awareness inward toward the breath and the self. Also, they work economically as preparations for both reclining and sitting pranayama.

PRELIMINARY

Read carefully through the description of each asana before you do it. As you read, imagine yourself doing the work, step-by-step, mentally rehearsing your actual performance. In this chapter's "Last Word," I'll suggest some ways to organize warm-up sequences and other practices with these postures.

Each of the asanas will focus on a particular bone or bony structure (that is, the sacrum, ribs, scapulas, and the sternum and clavicles) or body area (like the groins and belly). We've already had a look at most of the bony structures (in chapter 9). The groins are the creases between the thighs and pelvis. I'm dividing the groins into the inner groins, where the inner thighs join the base of the pelvis at the perineum, and the front groins, where the front thighs join the front pelvis.

The belly—which we usually associate with the word pot—is divided into the lower belly, from the pubis to the navel, and upper belly, from the navel to the bottom tip of the sternum.

Inner Groins: Reclining Bound Angle Posture (Supta Baddha Konasana)

Kona means "corner" or "angle," and *baddha* means "bound," "tied," "fettered." *Supta* means "lying down to sleep, though not actually asleep," and is usually translated as "reclining."

Tight groins are common among beginning students. There are several reasons why this is so, but one of the biggest culprits is chair sitting. It would be much healthier for our groins if we could all sit on the floor with our legs crossed while working at our computer or squat while waiting for the bus to come, but that's just not the way we do things in this culture. We'll come back to the issue of chair sitting in chapter 15.

What's the problem with tight groins, anyway? The groins are sort of right in the middle of things, and when they're tight, those things don't work as well. The energy that ideally flows freely out of the pelvis, up along the front spine through the crown, and down along the legs into the heels gets stuck. Then the spine can't lift and the heels can't ground, and we sag forward depressingly and can't stand on our own two feet. Tight groins also hamper the pumping action of the thoracic diaphragm, which makes everyday breathing a chore and pranayama nearly impossible.

In this first of two variations of Reclining Bound Angle, we'll open— or try to open, anyway—the gate of the inner groins. We'll turn our efforts to the front groins in the exercises that immediately follow.

PRACTICE: RECLINING BOUND ANGLE POSTURE 1

You'll need two blankets and two sandbags for this posture. Fold the two blankets widthwise five times. Lie on your back and, bending your knees to the sides, join the soles of your feet. Settle the outside edges of the feet on the floor and the heels at a comfortable distance from the pelvis. Position the blankets under your outer thighs, right in the crease where they join the pelvis, so that the sharp edges of the blankets are perpendicular to the thighbones. Support the legs a little higher than their maximum stretch. Lay the bags across the top inner thighs, parallel to the creases of the groins (see fig. 14.1).

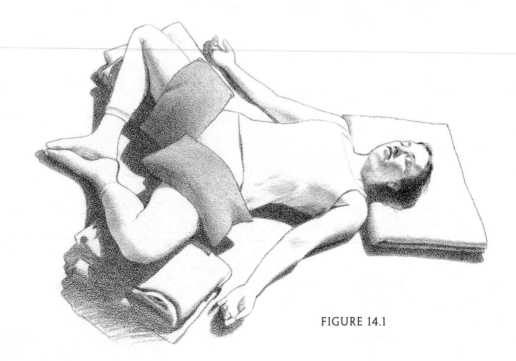

FIGURE 14.1

Stay in this position for anywhere from five to ten minutes.

To exit, slide the bags off the thighs toward the torso. Put your hands against the outer thighs and, with an exhale, press the thighs together, keeping the muscles of the inner thighs as soft as possible. Draw the knees into the abdomen, again with an exhale; wrap your hands around the shins or the backs of the thighs; and squeezing the thighs to the belly, press the lower back against the floor.

HOW IT HELPS

Reclining Bound Angle stretches the muscles of the inner thighs and groins and encourages the femur heads to center in the hip sockets. This creates space—the final frontier—and releases pelvic energy to ripple up along the front spine to the crown and down into the earth through the heels. Space in the groins also frees the thoracic and pelvic diaphragms and so makes breathing a joy.

Caution. Don't put the bags on your inner thighs without the blankets under the outer thighs. Don't push the knees toward the floor, which simply encourages the inner groins to harden. Imagine instead that your knees are floating up toward the ceiling.

GOING FURTHER

To increase the stretch, imagine that the bags are sinking into the thighs. At the same time, release the thighs away from the bags. Go on playing this little game—sinking the bags, then releasing the thighs—for as long as you stay in this posture.

Use your hands to push the outer thighs away from the sides of the torso. At the same time, draw the pubis closer to the navel, softening the lower belly. Press the outer heels together and the outer knees apart.

Front Groins

Here are two exercises for the front groins, Bent-Knee Lunge for beginners and Reclining Half Hero for more experienced students. If you're not familiar with these postures and unsure whether you're a beginner or more of an intermediate, go with Bent-Knee Lunge for a while and then carefully transition to the second exercise.

PRACTICE: BENT-KNEE LUNGE

For this exercise you'll need to go to your yoga wall with a strap and blanket. Fold the blanket widthwise three or four times, then kneel on it facing your yoga wall, an arm's length away. Step your left foot forward, touch your big toe to the wall, and position the knee directly over the ankle, so the shin is perpendicular to the floor. Exhale and slide the right knee back, keeping the left knee over the ankle, until you feel a comfortable stretch in the right front thigh and groin. Loop the buckled strap over your torso and snug it over the front knee and the back thigh, just below the crease of the buttock (see fig. 14.2).

Stay for an equal length of time on both sides. Come out of the lunge with an inhalation. Start with thirty seconds to a minute on each side and gradually work your way up to three minutes.

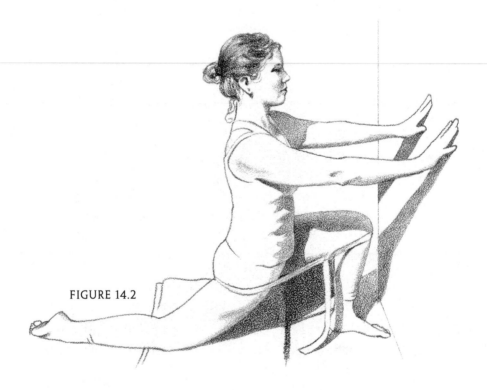

FIGURE 14.2

HOW IT HELPS

Bent-Knee Lunge stretches the muscles of the back leg's front thigh and groin, and the abdomen. It also helps center the heads of both femurs in their hip sockets. By pressing down on the sacrum and tailbone, as suggested in the following "Caution" section, you'll learn how to lengthen and deepen—or as Mr. Iyengar says, sharpen—the coccyx, a useful action in many asanas, especially back bends, and muscular locks (bandha, which we'll look at in chapter 20).

Caution. If your lower back hurts, lift the front knee out of the lunge slightly by drawing it a few inches away from the wall. With the same-side hand as the forward knee, push down actively on the tailbone, lengthening it toward the floor. At the same time, draw the pubis toward the navel. Maintain the angle of the pelvis relative to the floor, keep the hand in place on the tail, and drop the front knee over the ankle again. If, after this, the pain returns, repeat these instructions but also draw the back knee a few inches closer to the wall.

GOING FURTHER

Keep the front knee over the ankle and strongly press the back thigh against the strap. Imagine that the back-leg femur head is moving away from the wall but, at the same time, the same-side hip is pressing toward the wall, so that the front of your pelvis stays relatively parallel to the wall.

Be sure to press the tailbone down toward the floor and forward toward the wall, to lengthen the lower back. Push on the tailbone with a hand if you need help with this movement. Lift the pubis toward the navel.

PRACTICE: RECLINING HALF HERO (SUPTA ARDHA VIRASANA)

Vira means "brave or eminent man," "hero," "chief" (and with a long final a, it means "wife" or "matron"). It's distantly related to our words virtue and virile. *Ardha* means "half." This posture is a variation of Hero or Heroine (virasana), which we'll go into in chapter 16.

For this posture you'll need some support for your back, either a bolster or one or more blankets folded up to serve as a bolster. If you're tighter in the groins, you'll need a thicker bolster; with more open groins, you can use less support. But even if you can lie comfortably on the floor in this posture, I recommend that you have some support under your spine. You'll need at least one blanket, though, and you might also want a sandbag, a block, and a washcloth.

Sit on the floor with straight legs and position one end of the bolster against the back of your pelvis. Lean to your left, bend your right knee, and stand your right foot on the floor by the sitting bones (the two stirrup-shaped bones at the bottom of the pelvis). Grab onto the right ankle and, swinging the bent knee and shin down onto the floor, pull the right foot back beside the hip. Make sure the foot points straight back, not out to the right, and that the top of the foot is broad on the floor so there's as much pressure on the little-toe side of the foot as on the big-toe side. Raise the bent knee a few inches off the floor on a folded blanket, then lay the heavy bag across the top of the thigh, parallel to the crease of the front groin and directly over the femur head. Sit upright for a minute or two, to stretch the front thigh muscles. Then carefully lie back on your bolster. Your left leg can be straight or bent at the knee (see fig. 14.3).

Stay for an equal length of time on both sides. Start with thirty seconds to a minute and work your way up gradually to three to five minutes.

Be very careful of your knees when exiting either version of Hero, the half here or its full partner later on. Remember that your knees

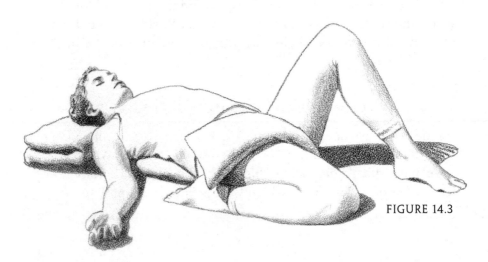

FIGURE 14.3

are hinge joints that don't do well with any kind of rotary movement, which should always be centered in your hip joints.

To extricate yourself here, lift off the support with an exhale to sitting, leading with the sternum and trailing the head. Take the sandbag off the thigh. Then push your hands on the floor on either side of your hips and lift your buttocks away from the floor. Slide the Half Hero foot under the lifted buttocks so the knee swings out to the side, then sit back down on the floor. Your heel will be tucked into the perineum and your outer leg will be on the floor. Slowly straighten the bent leg out to the side, then swing it back straight in front of you from the hip. Bounce the knee up and down on the floor a few times.

HOW IT HELPS

If you're not used to Reclining Half Hero, you may wonder at first how it will ever be of help to you. In my beginning classes, this posture regularly ranks among the top five in the "Most Contorted" category—usually accompanied by some of the most agonized faces you'll ever see. That's why it's recommended that you start with the Bent-Knee Lunge before you tackle Reclining Half Hero.

But over time this posture can actually become a relaxing position—trust me here—as it stretches the muscles of the front thigh, groin, and abdomen and helps center the femur head in the hip socket, all of which will help your breathing immensely.

Caution. There are several things to be aware of in this posture. For starters, many beginning students have some pain in the fronts of the ankles on the Half Hero leg. If you have this problem, roll up a washcloth and wedge it underneath the ankle. That should lessen the discomfort somewhat.

Beginners also find that the Half Hero knee wants to slide out to the right, beyond the line of the hip joint. As you see from the above practice instructions, I want you to have your Half Hero knee elevated slightly off the floor, which helps the sandbag sink deeper into the groin, but I don't want the knee to angle outside the line of the hip. If you run up against this problem, firm the inner thigh and draw the knee back toward the midline. If, despite your best efforts, the bent-knee leg keeps sliding out, squeeze a block between the bent knee and the inner foot of the free leg.

Then there's the matter of your lower back. If it feels jammed, use your hands to press the back of your pelvis toward the tailbone and imagine that the tail is spooling out along the floor, like one of those steel tape rulers. If that doesn't work, add one or more blankets to your bolster. Find a bolster height that gets you a good stretch on the Half Hero leg yet allows your back to lengthen comfortably.

There are some knee and back problems that could be exacerbated by this posture. If you have chronic pain in either or both of these areas, talk with an experienced teacher before attempting this posture. As an alternative, work with the Bent-Knee Lunge, described earlier in the chapter.

GOING FURTHER

Be aware of the top of the right thigh, just below the weight. The front groin is a shallow crease between the front of the pelvis and the thigh. Imagine that the bag is sinking deeper into this crease and pressing the femur head deeper into the hip socket. Neither the bag nor the bone will ever hit bottom—as long as you stay in the posture, both will continue to slowly drop toward the floor.

Sacrum

PRACTICE: RECLINING BOUND ANGLE POSTURE 2 (SUPTA BADDHA KONASANA)

This posture is similar in form to the first Reclining Bound Angle, but it has a different intent. In the earlier version we wanted to open the groins; here we'll learn a little about the proper movement of the sacrum so that we can eventually apply the lesson to our sitting position.

You'll need a block and, if you need to pad the block, a sticky mat or towel. Lie on your back, knees bent, feet on the floor. Inhale, lift the pelvis away from the floor, and slide the block under the sacrum with the faces of the block parallel to the floor and its long axis parallel to your spine. Exhale down onto the block, join your soles, and drop your knees to the sides. If the block feels too hard against your sacrum, use a folded sticky mat or a towel as a pad. I have various-sized pieces of old sticky mat in my practice room to use as pads (see fig. 14.4).

Now with the thumbs against the inner thighs and the fingers splayed on the outer, grip the tops of your thighs just where they join the pelvis. Firmly rotate the thighs outward, so that the outer thighs lengthen away from the sides of your torso. Then stroke your hands out along the outer thighs from the hips to the knees.

Finally, hook your hands underneath the hip points on the front of the pelvis. Push them together toward the navel and pull them up toward your shoulders. These actions will help protect your lower back and open your inner groins.

Stay in this position anywhere from three to five minutes.

To exit, spread your hands against the outer thighs and, with an exhale, press the thighs together, keeping the muscles of the inner thighs as soft as possible. Stand the feet on the floor, inhale the pelvis off the block, slide the block to one side, and finally exhale and roll the spine, from the highest vertebra that's off the floor to the tail, down onto the floor. Draw the knees into the abdomen, again with an exhale; wrap your hands around the shins or the backs of the thighs; and squeezing the thighs to the belly, press the lower back against the floor.

HOW IT HELPS

The rocking and scrubbing of the sacrum on the block, and the pressure of the block against the sacrum, teaches the three basic movements of the sacrum. Like the first variation earlier in the chapter, this second one stretches the muscles of the inner thighs and groins.

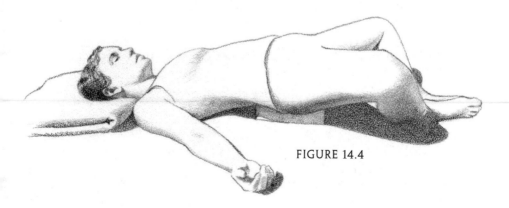

FIGURE 14.4

Caution. If, despite the actions described above in the "Practice" section, you still feel pain in your lower back, the first thing to do is to press your thumbs against the end of the block, as if you were—but not actually—pushing it away from the back of your torso. This should help to further lengthen the lower spine. If it doesn't, then lie at a lower height. You could also stay at the same height but raise your feet a few inches off the ground on a folded blanket.

GOING FURTHER

Rock to the right. Feel the edge of the block press up against the right side of your sacrum. At the same time, without pushing the knee down, release the inner thigh toward the floor. Imagine that the right sacrum is lifting while the inner thigh descends. Rock slowly back and forth from right to left several times, imagining that the sacrum is widening as you do. Gradually diminish the rocking action until you're resting evenly on the block.

Then push the outer edges of the feet lightly against the floor. Without actually sliding off the block, feel the block scrub down on the sacrum, drawing its head toward the tailbone.

If you're relatively comfortable lying on the face of the block and want to increase your challenge, inhale, lift your pelvis up, and spin the block onto one of its sides. Lie back down with an exhale. Recreate the same actions that you did at the lower height.

If you're still comfortable on the sides of the block—and this is for experienced students only—inhale and again lift the pelvis up. Here you may need to put the feet on the floor and push up into a Bridge-like position first, just to get the block in place. Turn the block now onto one of its ends and lie back down with an exhale. Careful, though—this is a real stretch.

Hips: Auspicious Posture (Svastikasana)

A svastika is any lucky or auspicious object, but especially a cross or mark made on persons to denote good luck. Svastikasana is usually described as a simple cross-legged posture, similar to the Easy posture (sukhasana, described in chapter 16). I'm applying the name here to a kind of loose cross-legged position.

Most beginning students are very tight around the hips, though this is probably more true for males than females. This tightness affects the openness of our groins as well as our capacity to sit properly for pranayama.

There are two variations of the Auspicious posture, the first for beginning asana students, the second for intermediates.

PRACTICE: AUSPICIOUS POSTURE—VARIATION 1

In order for this posture to have its most auspicious effects, you'll need a blanket and block. Sit on the edge of the blanket that's been folded three or four times widthwise, knees bent at right angles, feet on the floor. Cross the legs at the shins, so that each foot is below the opposite thigh. Exhale and lean forward; rest your forehead on the block. Find a height that lets you lean forward comfortably in this position (see fig.14.5).

Stay for two to three minutes, then repeat, with the left shin crossed in front of the right.

Caution. If you're tighter in the hips or groins, you may find even this simple cross-legged sitting position a challenge. The first thing to do is raise yourself on a higher support by adding one or more folded blankets to your base or sit on a round bolster. If this still doesn't help, then open the cross of the legs a bit by unbending the knees slightly and sliding the feet away from the pelvis.

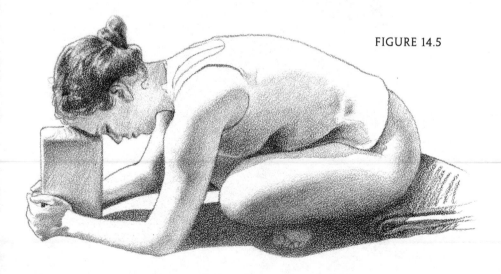

FIGURE 14.5

If you lean forward to rest your head on the block and find your back or neck straining and the front of your torso collapsing, then be sure to get a higher support for your head, like the seat of a chair.

PRACTICE: AUSPICIOUS POSTURE—VARIATION 2

Sit on the edge of the blanket folded three or four times widthwise, knees bent at right angles, feet on the floor. Slide the left foot under the right leg, position it just beside the right hip, and lay the outside of the leg on the floor. Cross the right leg over the left and position the right ankle just to the outside of the left knee, with the sole perpendicular to the floor (see fig. 14.6).

Put your left hand on the floor, lean over to that side, and lift your right buttock an inch or two off the blanket. Burrow your right thumb deep into the inner right groin, then slowly release the right buttock back to the blanket. Sit upright or, if you want to increase the stretch in the hip, exhale and lean slightly forward, pressing the hands on the floor in front of you. You can also twist, either from the upright or from the forward lean, toward the top-leg side.

Stay for two to three minutes, then repeat, with the left leg crossed on top of the right.

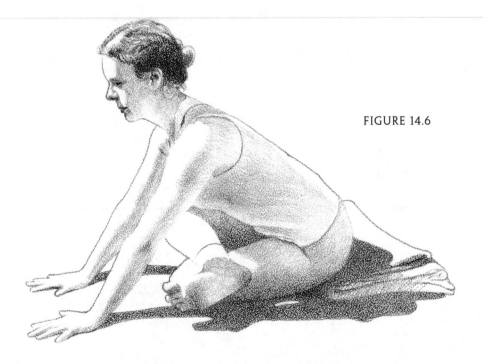

FIGURE 14.6

HOW IT HELPS

Auspicious posture, especially in its intermediate version, is another one of those postures that students love to . . . if not exactly hate, then to grumble and groan about. As most students quickly discover, it's a wonderful stretch for the hips and groins. It works best if it's held for several minutes—though the temptation is to quit the position after only a few seconds—while breathing deeply into the pelvis.

Caution. To protect the top knee, it's important to have the top ankle outside the bottom knee and the sole of the top foot perpendicular, not parallel, to the floor.

GOING FURTHER

Imagine that, from the center of the sacrum, you're pushing the knees away from the pelvis. Watch, then, how the sacrum fans across the back of the pelvis as it feeds into the knees.

Belly

The long vertical muscle of the front belly (rectus abdominis), which stretches between the pubis and sternum, is the diaphragm's breathing synergist. That's a fancy way of saying that the two muscles act cooperatively to pump air into and out of the body. I won't go into the boring details: suffice it to say that when one of this pair is contracting, the other is releasing—at least, that's the ideal.

We tend, though, to hold a lot of unnecessary tension in our bellies. This tension prevents the diaphragm from working properly, which naturally affects both our everyday breathing and our pranayama.

PRACTICE: BELLY ROLL

The name of this exercise may suggest that we're going to roll around on our belly. While this sounds like a lot of fun, and might actually serve some useful purpose, what we're really going to do is lie faceup with a roll under our belly—or to be more precise, under the natural curve of our lower back. So you'll need a blanket roll or a small round bolster, like a pranayama bolster. You could also use a folded blanket to support and pad the back of your head. Your roll, whether it's a rolled-up blanket or a bolster, should fit comfortably into the normal curve of your lower back. Lie down with the roll under your lower back and keep your knees bent and feet on the floor. You can either rest your arms out to the sides, palms up, or put your fingertips on your lower belly, below the navel. Use the second blanket, if necessary, to support the back of your head.

Release the lower spine completely onto the roll. Press the tailbone toward the heels, lift the pubis toward the navel, and slide the lower back ribs away from the roll. (see fig. 14.7)

You can keep your knees bent throughout the entire exercise or extend your legs, one at a time, pushing out from the hip through the heel. If you do this, though, keep the legs and feet active, pressing the inner thighs to the floor and stretching the balls of the feet to the ceiling.

You can also work the arms. Raise the arms perpendicular to the floor and cross the forearms, holding the elbows with your hands. Push the elbows toward the ceiling to charge the arms and then, with an inhale, swing the arms overhead. Extend strongly through the elbows and heels.

Stay in this position for five minutes or more.

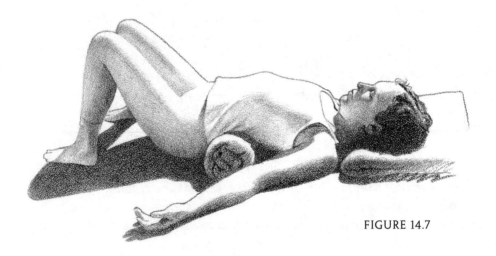

FIGURE 14.7

HOW IT HELPS

Belly Roll stretches the rectus abdominis and over time will help release tension in your belly. The imaginary actions of the pelvis and the weight, along with the lifted groins, will slightly hollow your lower belly, a condition we'll return to (in chapter 20) when we go into abdominal control.

Caution. Be sure not to poke the lower front ribs up toward the ceiling and harden the muscles along the lower spine. Soften the lower back muscles and spread them on the roll.

GOING FURTHER

Turn over and lie prone on the roll. Support your head on your crossed forearms and turn your toes inward. Wedge the roll between your lower ribs and the top rim of your pelvis, right into the soft area of the belly. On the inhales lift your upper torso slightly by pushing the forearms against the floor and lengthen the lower ribs away from the roll. At the same time, press your tail toward your heels to anchor the back spine. Then on the exhales release the lift and sink your belly more deeply over the roll.

Ribs: Revolved Belly Posture (Jathara Parivartanasana) —Bent-Knee Variation

Jathara means "belly"; *parivartana* means "to turn around," "to revolve." This is a modified version of the full posture, in which the legs are extended and the feet directed toward the outstretched hands.

Although the name of this posture refers to the belly, and I've headed this section "Ribs," what we're really up to here is stretching the muscles between the ribs, the intercostals. Though the diaphragm is the workhorse breathing muscle—I read somewhere once that it's responsible for up to 70 percent of quiet breathing—there are other muscles, like the intercostals, that lend a hand in everyday breathing. Because we're inclined to slouch under the collective weight of modern civilization, these muscles often are very tight, which hinders our breathing more than it helps.

PRACTICE: REVOLVED BELLY POSTURE—BENT-KNEE VARIATION

For this exercise you'll need one or two blankets. Lie on your back and, with an exhale, draw your knees up to your torso. Take some time to hug the thighs against the abdomen, pressing the back against the floor. Then release the legs and twist them, on an exhale, to the left until the outer left leg rests on the floor. Turn the upper torso to the right. Place the left hand on the outer right knee and gently press the knees to the floor; at the same time, stretch the right arm away from the torso, parallel to the top line of the shoulders (see fig. 14.8).

To exit, exhale and lift the legs back to the starting position. You can lift one leg at a time or, for more of a challenge, both at the same time.

Twist to each side of the posture for an equal length of time, from one to three minutes.

HOW IT HELPS

Along with the intercostals, Revolved Belly posture stretches the side abdominal muscles, the oblique. It massages organs like the liver and spleen as well as the intestines.

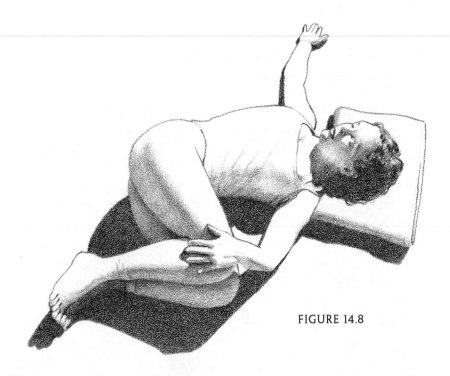

FIGURE 14.8

Caution. When the legs are twisted to the left, the right shoulder often doesn't rest easily on the floor (the same is true of the left shoulder when the legs are twisted to the right). Don't force this shoulder down. Instead, lift the opposite shoulder slightly away from the floor and then extend more actively through the raised shoulder's arm.

Beginning asana students should keep the head in a neutral position, looking straight up at the ceiling. Intermediates can turn the head to look at the straight arm.

If there's any pain in your lower back, work with the downward release of the spine through the tailbone. If the pain persists, raise the legs on a thickly folded blanket or bolster.

GOING FURTHER

In the twist the top ribs often bulge out of the torso while the bottom ribs lift into the torso. This indicates that the spine is not lengthening evenly from side to side, which restricts the twist. Reach across with the opposite-side hand and draw the top ribs into the torso. When both sides of the torso feel equally long, return the hand to the top knee, pull the knee away from the pelvis, and open yourself diagonally from the knees through the straight arm.

Touch the thumb of the hand toward which your upper torso is twisting to the highest vertebra you can reach. Press the bony knob of the bone down toward the tailbone and into the torso. Continue down the back of the spine, pushing each little bump down and in; cross the sacrum; and lengthen out along the tailbone.

Scapulas: Couch Posture (Paryankasana) —Supported Variation

A paryanka is a bed, couch, sofa. The full posture is performed with the legs in Hero posture, no block support under the scapulas, and the crown of the head on the floor, but we won't try that here. If you're curious about what it looks like, see the photo in *Light on Yoga*.

You're probably used to sitting on couches with nice, soft cushions. Don't be misled by the name of this posture. Here you'll be arching your torso in such a way that—if you squint your eyes and use your imagination—you'll look like a couch. Just as we learned earlier about the movements of the sacrum in preparation for sitting, here we'll learn about the movements of the scapulas in the sitting position.

PRACTICE: COUCH POSTURE—SUPPORTED VARIATION

I'll describe two different ways to support your back. For the first way you'll need a block, and if you need to pad it to protect your back, a folded sticky mat or towel. If you prefer the second way, you'll need a blanket rolled up to about a five- to six-inch diameter.

Some students like the firmness—or you might say the definitiveness—of the block support, which can be bare or padded with a folded sticky mat.

Set the block on the floor, resting on one of its faces, and lie on it so that its long axis is perpendicular to your spine. Make sure your scapulas are completely supported. You can either lie on the bare block or, if you find that uncomfortable, pad the block with a folded blanket or sticky mat. Begin practicing this exercise with your knees bent and feet on the floor, and your arms comfortably out to your sides, angled about 45 degrees to the torso. After a minute or so, if you like, you can raise your arms overhead, as the model is showing here (see fig. 14.9). You can either keep your arms straight, palms facing the ceiling, or clasp your bent elbows with your hands. Whether straight or bent though, be sure not to force the arms to the floor, which will harden the shoulders and front torso. Other students would rather lie on a bed of nails than on the block. If you

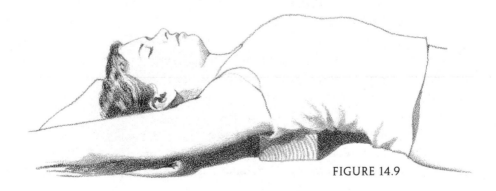

FIGURE 14.9

find the block uncomfortable even after it's been padded, then lie on a rolled-up blanket instead. Fold the blanket widthwise twice, so that it measures about two feet by three feet. Hold one of the long edges in your hands and roll the blanket up into a thin, firm roll. Start by lying on the roll so that it's below your upper shoulder blades. Push your feet against the floor and slide over the roll until it's just below the lower tips of your scapulas.

With either one of these supports, if your head doesn't rest comfortably on the floor, raise it up on a folded blanket. Now raise your arms perpendicular to the floor. Push the inner border of the right scapula away from the spine and extend the right arm toward the ceiling. Do the same on the left. Go back and forth a few times, from right to left, reaching up toward the ceiling by widening the scapulas. Then, maintaining the width across your back, return the arms to the floor.

Push your feet against the floor. Without actually sliding off the block or the roll, feel the block push the scapulas toward the tailbone. Imagine that, as the front torso drapes over the block, the scapulas are lifting into the torso.

Stay for three to five minutes.

HOW IT HELPS

Couch teaches the three essential movements of the scapulas, which we'll eventually apply to our sitting position, and stretches the intercostal muscles.

It's also a powerful heart opener. Many of us spend parts or most of our working days leaning forward over a desk or hunched over a steering wheel driving a car to and from work. This tends over time to collapse the upper chest and block the upper tips of the lungs, making everyday breathing a chore. You can easily see this for yourself in the people around you every day, at the office, on the street, even in yoga class. If this sounds like you, then Couch is a posture you'll want to do regularly and often to pry open some space in the upper chest.

Caution. Couch isn't always a comfortable position, either physically or psychologically. As we've been discovering as we wend our way through the exercises and up along the body, we have areas of tension that, when disturbed, can kick back with varying degrees of displeasure.

Though ostensibly we're working on the proper movement of the scapulas, as I've mentioned, Couch also serves to stretch the heart area. I've seen some interesting reactions to this position in my classes over the years. Some students have trouble breathing; others melt into a puddle of tears. While it's useful to push the limits of your capacity, it's rarely a good idea to force yourself beyond them. The lions, elephants, and tigers would advise you to go slowly with Couch. If the height of either the block or the blanket roll seems as if it's too much to bear, then immediately find yourself a lower support, either by moving from the block to the roll or by unrolling the blanket slightly to reduce its diameter. Always breathe deeply and smoothly into your heart, using your breath to soften the area around the sternum.

GOING FURTHER

As you did with the Belly Roll, you can keep your knees bent in Couch, or you can extend your legs, one at a time, pushing out from the hip through the heel. Again, keep the legs and feet active, pressing the inner thighs to the floor and stretching the balls of the feet to the ceiling.

You can also work the arms as you did before in the Belly Roll. Raise the arms perpendicular to the floor, then cross the forearms, hold the elbows with the opposite hands, then swing the crossed arms overhead with an inhale. Don't expect the forearms to drop easily to the floor and don't force them to the floor if they don't. Bring the forearms overhead just until you feel the front ribs begin to poke up toward the ceiling. At this point stop the movement, raise the forearms an inch, release the front torso, then lower the forearms slightly. Be patient. As the muscles of the armpits release, the forearms will sink toward the floor.

Extend strongly through the elbows and heels.

Sternum and Clavicles: Bridge Posture (Setu Bandhasana)—Supported Variation

A setu is "something that binds or fetters," like a dike or dam, which, if you think about it, binds water. It also means "bridge." Setubandha is "the forming of a causeway or bridge." Look at a picture of this posture (fig. 14.10) from the side on, and you'll quickly see the rationale for the name.

PRACTICE: BRIDGE POSTURE—SUPPORTED VARIATION

For this exercise use two blankets or a round bolster and, optionally, a strap and block. Fold each blanket widthwise twice. Then fold each blanket lengthwise in thirds; that is, fold the blanket over twice so that it's one-third of its original width. Then stack the two blankets, sharp edges matching. You can use more blankets if you want a higher support.

Sit on the middle of the blankets with your back toward the sharp edge, knees bent and feet on the floor to either side of the support. Exhale and lie back onto the blankets with your head just at the sharp edge. Exhale again, push your feet against the floor, and slowly slide over the sharp edge of the blankets, so that it pulls down on the back of your torso and scapulas. Stop when the tops of your shoulders lightly touch the floor. The sharp edge of the blankets will be somewhere between your scapulas, at what I call the root of the neck. Stretch your arms out to the sides, palms up (see fig.14.10).

Keep the knees bent or, if you like, straighten your legs onto the support. My heels hang over the dull edge of the blankets, so I support them on the face of a block. If you straighten your legs, you can bind them together with a strap positioned just above the knees.

Stay for five to ten minutes.

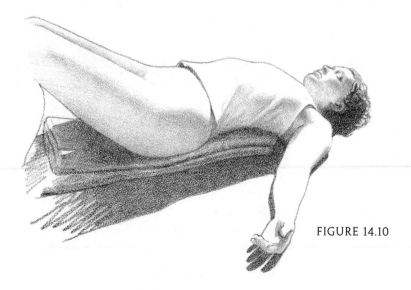

FIGURE 14.10

HOW IT HELPS

Like the Couch, Bridge lifts and opens the heart and frees the breath in the upper lungs. It stretches the front armpits (pectoralis major), the back of the neck, and the front of the torso and thighs and strengthens the muscles of the back spine.

Bridge is an excellent preparation for Net-Bearer Lock (jaland-hara-bandha, which we'll look at in chapter 20).

Caution. Most students will encourage the opening of their chest in this posture with two actions: forcefully pulling the tops of their shoulders away from the ears and squeezing their scapulas together toward the spine. Neither action, though, is a good idea.

Pulling the shoulders away from the ears will overstretch the muscles of the back of the neck and lead to some painful results. Instead, as you perform this posture, lift the shoulders slightly toward the ears. Then broaden the scapulas and press them firmly against the back torso, as if you were still lying on the block in Couch. Press the heads of the humerus bones down on the floor.

By the same token, never force the chin toward the sternum. Lift the chin slightly away from the chest and boost the sternum toward the chin from the lift of the scapulas.

GOING FURTHER

Imagine that you're lifting the root of the neck in two directions: up toward the crown of your head and diagonally through your torso to the top of the sternum. Be careful, as you create this latter action, not to help it along by pushing the lower front ribs up toward the ceiling. As you lift the manubrium by firming the scapulas against the back, release the xiphoid down toward the navel.

PLAYING AROUND: DYNAMIC BENT-KNEE LUNGE

If you think about my descriptions of the nine postures, you'll find a common thread running through them, which is that they're all held statically. If you're an experienced asana student, then there's a good chance that this is the way you've been trained in your classes to perform the asanas—no less an authority than Patanjali himself maintains that a successful asana must be steady and comfortable. Then each time you practice the asana, you try to re-create some ideal form, which never changes.

But is this the only way to execute these positions? Some teachers would answer this question with a resounding "No!" They believe that the original yoga asanas weren't fixed positions at all; instead, they were ec-static (literally "out of stationariness") expressions of Goddess energy (lila) surging through the bodies of her devotees. Each asana was a rhythmic dance that was never repeated. Over the centuries, these teachers contend, these wavelike shapes crystallized into the static postures we know today.

Of course, I'm not advocating here that we all abandon the traditional forms. But we can inject something of the asana's wild and crazy origins into our work. Let's take our simple Bent-Knee Lunge and play with it a little. It will give you a feel for this more improvisational approach and perhaps sow the seeds for other playful experiments with the asanas.

You'll need to go back to your yoga wall with a blanket. Set yourself up as before at your yoga wall, kneeling on a blanket (we won't use the strap here as we did for the stationary posture). Again step your left foot forward, touch your big toe to the wall, and position the knee directly over the ankle, so the shin is perpendicular to the floor. Exhale and slide the right knee back, keeping the left knee over the ankle, until you feel a comfortable stretch in the right-front thigh and groin.

This time, though, don't hold the lunge statically. Begin to move as the inner spirit urges you, maybe rocking back and forth on the right knee or swaying your hips left and right or reaching your hands high up on the wall and then sweeping them to one side or the other to lengthen the sides of the torso. I can't instruct you here how to be spontaneous and playful. The important thing to remember is, don't think about what you're doing, just let your body move. Your movements can be rhythmic and regular or arrhythmic and irregular, never repeated a second time, large and expressive or small and subtle.

Then you can continue to play throughout your entire stay in the posture, or you can gradually slow your movements down until you stop and hold the posture—whatever you feel inspired to do. Try to work for more or less equal lengths of time on both sides.

HOW IT HELPS

For me playfulness in asana breaks down habitual barriers and goal seeking in my body-mind and suggests new possibilities for movement and feeling. I momentarily step out of the confines of the traditional form and authority and call on the wisdom of my own inner voice for guidance.

GOING FURTHER

Just about any asana lends itself to playfulness, though some more than others. It's easy, for example, to play around with two-feet-on-the-ground postures like Mountain (tadasana) or Triangle (trikonasana) but less so with balancing postures like Tree (vrikshasana) or Headstand (shirshasana). There's no right way to play with an asana. Let your spirit be your guide. Just remember that all of the safety rules regarding things like knees and necks still apply.

LAST WORD

You can practice these postures in preparation for pranayama in one of two ways. You can focus on just one area of your body, like your groins or ribs, and choose postures that work that area or at least work that area primarily. Or alternatively you can do a general preparation and choose a range of postures that work just about every part of you.

How long you practice, of course, depends on how much time you have available. Ideally you should try to do some preparation for every breathing session—say, five to ten minutes—but this may not always be possible. If I'm rushed for time, I like to lie in Couch or Bridge for a few minutes, just to open the area around my heart.

How many of these postures you do again depends on your available time. There are two ways to go about filling up your prep time: do more postures, holding each for the minimum time suggested, or do fewer postures but hold each for the maximum time suggested or even longer.

You can order the postures in different ways. I've listed them in the chapter in one possible practice sequence. You can also change the postures you practice from day to day, or you can stay with one or the same group of postures for a while—say, a week or ten days.

Remember that the nine postures aren't the only good preparations for pranayama. There are lots more. Ask your teacher or look in other guidebooks for more ideas about what to practice. Also remember that these postures aren't meant as a substitute for a regular asana practice.

CHAPTER 15

Chair Seat

When a man has found this correct centre of gravity in
his body he can open himself to the forces that lie at the
essential core of life and anchor himself therein. . . .
When he is relaxed and firmly based in this centre man
experiences these forces in his physical existence. . . . It is
the centre of gravity which determines the total posture
of the body as well as its patterns of tension and the character of its breathing.

—Karlfried Graf Von Durckheim, *The Way of Transformation*

I DON'T KNOW about you, but I spend a large chunk of my day sitting at my computer hunting and pecking away at my keyboard.
Most of us probably don't think a lot about how much we sit and the
way we typically sit every day, but we really should. Faulty chair
design, the prevalence of chair sitting, and our lack of understanding of how to sit properly—a kind of sitting avidya—have lately been
singled out as major contributors to poor posture and the conse-
quent ubiquity of back problems in our culture.

Sometimes I think it would be easier if we could just always lie
down for our practice. Cradled supine in the gravity field, there's
so much less to worry about than when sitting. But eventually we
have to get up off our back and sit. This, of course, completely
changes our relationship to gravity, and any imbalances in our posture are quickly revealed and experienced as physical obstacles.
After a few misaligned minutes in an unaccustomed sitting position,
especially with an unsupported back and crossed legs, the average
beginning breather, unless he's had some experience sitting in meditation, starts to squirm and sink. This is quite the opposite of Patanjali's injunction that our asana be steady and comfortable. Then
pranayama is nearly impossible.

Just as pranayama breathing is different from everyday breathing, so is pranayama sitting different from everyday sitting. In this chapter we'll focus on what I think of as the fundamental pranayama seat, a phrase suggested by the Durckheim quote. The word fundamental comes to us from two Latin words, fundare, "to lay the foundation," and fundus, "bottom." Fundamental sitting lays the foundation for pranayama sitting and is appropriately built upward from the bottom of the pelvis, the sitting bones.

The bad news, at least for those of you looking forward to finally sitting in a traditional seat for pranayama, is that we're not quite ready to do that yet. This is the lions, elephants, and tigers approach, remember, and we never do anything straightforwardly. It makes little sense at the outset of sitting practice, given our sitting avidya, to adopt a traditional seat. In fundamental sitting we'll take up residence in a decidedly untraditional seat—a chair—as a transition stage between reclining and the more demanding floor sitting.

I know what you're thinking: if chair sitting is such a big problem in our culture, what in the world are we doing sitting in a chair for pranayama? Since we're all already seasoned chair sitters, chair sitting at the start of our sitting practice will grease the wheels of our transition. Used intelligently, the much-maligned chair can also help us master balanced sitting and liberate us from our sitting avidya. Naturally we'll be sitting on and, I suppose you could say, with the chair in entirely new ways. I've ingeniously named our revolutionary chair-sitting position Chair Seat.

Chair Seat

Mr. Iyengar briefly describes this seat in *Light on Pranayama* (see his chapter 11, "The Art of Sitting in Pranayama") as an alternative for students who can't, for various reasons, such as a knee injury, sit comfortably on the floor. But we'll use the chair here as a prop for our formal practice, regardless of our floor-sitting abilities.

There are two basic variations of the Chair Seat, back supported and unsupported. The latter variation is exactly the same as the former, save that your back isn't braced by the bolster and the wall. If you're brand new to sitting practice, or have some problems with your back or neck, then you might want to work with the supported variation first. Use your asana practice to strengthen your back—back bends are just the ticket for this—and gradually make the change to unsupported sitting.

PRELIMINARY

Metal folding chairs are a staple in Iyengar-style yoga classes. They're used not only for pranayama sitting but also as general asana supports, for standing postures; back bends; inverted positions, like supported head and shoulder stands; even occasionally for sitting, but only if you're stretching something, not for taking it easy. You'll need a suitable chair, a rolled-up sticky mat, a strap, and one or more sandbags. If you're sitting in the back-supported Chair Seat, you'll need a round bolster or rolled-up blanket. Set yourself up about a foot or so from your yoga wall, with your back to the wall.

Optional props include a blanket and a couple of blocks or a telephone book.

When you feel you're just about ready to move from reclining to Chair Seat, sit on your chair for five to ten minutes near the end of your asana practice or end your reclining practice and precede Corpse with a few minutes in Chair Seat. You could also sit for a few minutes in Chair Seat now and again throughout your day, when you have a quiet moment, just to reinforce what you're practicing.

During this preliminary period, sit on the front edge of your chair seat, hands resting softly on your thighs, eyes closed. Take a few minutes just to witness your sitting behavior. Try not to adjust yourself in any way; just sit as you typically do and observe. What would you say about the question Who is the sitter?

Of course, even though I've asked you not to adjust yourself, there's a good chance you'll be on your best sitting behavior. So for the first week or so of your transition to Chair Seat, try to witness your sitting behavior at odd moments during your day—at your desk, as you drive around in your car, or as you watch TV in the evening.

Don't worry too much about your breathing when you start with Chair Seat. Your first order of business is to understand how to sit in a steady and comfortable position. Next turn your Witness to the everyday breath and explore the four qualities again and, if needed, repeat the unusual-breathing exercises. Who's the breather now? What happens to the breather when he flips himself upright in the gravity field? Record your observations in your journal.

PRACTICE

Make sure you have the strap, the bag, the sticky mat, and the bolster handy before you sit through the chair. If you like, pad the chair seat with a folded blanket. Slide your legs through the space between the chair back and the seat. Next, slide yourself and the chair back against your yoga wall so the front edge of the seat is touching the wall. Lean forward slightly and wiggle the round bolster down between the channel of your spine and the wall, until its bottom rests on the chair seat. Then lean back. The bolster should touch your sacrum and the space between your scapulas but not your lower back or the back of your head. Now you'll be able to sit for a good long time (see fig. 15.1).

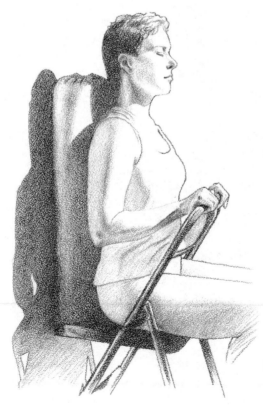

FIGURE 15.1

Roll the sticky mat up lengthwise and wedge it between your lower belly and the two chair legs. Arrange the thighs parallel to each other and the heels directly below the knees. If you have difficulty keeping your thighs parallel, snug the strap around them just above the knees, much as you did for the first variation of Bent-Knee Corpse. If you like, lay a sandbag or two across your top thighs. If you're shorter and your feet don't rest comfortably on the floor, put a block under each foot or a telephone book under both feet (see fig. 15.2).

Pelvis and Thighs

Your sitting bones are shaped like the curved rockers of a rocking chair. Rock your pelvis on these rockers. Rest your hands on the top rim of the pelvis to better feel the movement. Experiment with the

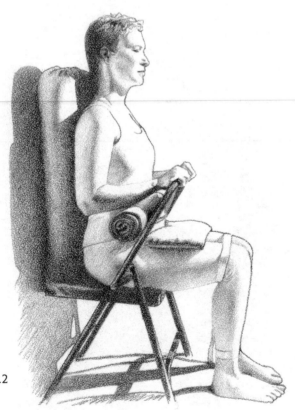

FIGURE 15.2

rhythm of the breath. For several breaths rock forward with the inhale and backward with the exhale. Then reverse for a few breaths.

Choose a rhythm that suits you and rock to and fro for a minute or so, leaning well forward and back. Gradually diminish the rocking action and come to a stop just a little forward of the midpoint of the sitting bones, where the top rim of the pelvis is parallel to the chair seat and the pubis and the tailbone are equidistant from the chair seat.

This is where you'll want to be when you sit both on the chair and on the floor. If you find that it's difficult to get forward on your sitting bones, that your pelvis insists on tipping backward, then raise your sitting bones on a folded sticky mat or blanket. Then work to stretch your hamstrings during your asana practice.

Sink the top thighs away from the heavy bag and feel the back thighs press firmly against the back edge of the seat. Imagine, as this happens, that the sitting bones are floating lightly away from the seat, so that you seem to be sitting more solidly on the backs of your thighs than on your sitting bones. Push the knees away from the hips, into the strap.

Shoulder Yoke

Hold the chair legs just below the chair back. Pull the legs down toward the floor and try to pull them apart—you can't, of course, and if you could, you would wreck your chair. This action of the hands will help you lower and broaden the shoulder blades. Spread the sternum into the clavicles and the clavicles away from the sternum. Remember that the shoulder yoke hangs from the back of the skull and sits on the top of the sternum, where it joins with the clavicles.

Spine

In yoga the spine is called the staff (danda) or the staff of Meru (meru-danda). This is a reference to the mythic golden mountain, Mount Meru, at the hub of the Hindu universe. Just as everything in the world rotates around Meru, so does our miniature world rotate around our spine.

The spine supplies structural support for the body-mind and the breath. A spine that is steady and comfortable encourages deep and easy breathing, and such breathing, in turn, lends additional support to the spine.

Imagine that your sacrum is pressing lightly and evenly into the pelvis, away from the strap. Be sure to soften the lower belly to receive this action. As you lengthen the back spine down through the coccyx, and the coccyx through the chair seat, lift your front spine through the crown of your head.

Then keep your spine very active. When the average person sits, he usually slouches so that the front of his spine is shorter than the back spine. In pranayama sitting the front of the spine lifts without hardening the back spine or pushing the front ribs forward. This makes the front of the body slightly longer than the back.

Head

There are two little bony bumps (occipital condyles) on the bottom of your skull that sit in two small indentations in the atlas. These are the sitting bones of your skull, like a pair of rockers on a rocking chair. Slowly nod "yes, yes, yes" on these rockers. Be sure that you're moving only from the rockers and that you keep the neck steady. Continue for a few minutes, slowly decreasing the nodding until you come to rest with the head in a neutral position. Imagine the head is floating on the top of the spine.

HOW IT HELPS

If you're not yet trained to sit for long periods in a traditional cross-legged seat, you'll have a much easier time getting through your practice in Chair Seat. It wards off numbness in the legs and feet and an aching back.

Sitting frees the movement of the back ribs, which are somewhat restricted by the reclining support. It also expands and intensifies our awareness of our body-mind.

Because of the position of the feet, legs, and hips, Chair Seat helps us sit up near the fronts of the sitting bones and so balance the pelvis, rib case, and head in the gravity field. This, in turn, allows us to lengthen the spine, which frees the diaphragm.

Chair Seat is a preparation not only for pranayama sitting but also for everyday chair sitting as we go about our daily business. At the very least, it's harder to fall asleep while sitting—although I have one student who is quite good at snoozing sitting up.

Caution. Chair Seat is a fairly easy position to assume; that's why I've chosen it to begin our sitting practice. But just as in Corpse and in the supported reclining positions, getting your balance established in Chair Seat can be a problem. Be sure that your sitting bones and upper back thighs are sitting evenly on the seat and that you're not leaning to one side or the other. See that your coccyx and pubis are equidistant from the seat or, as another way of measuring the same balance, that the top rim of your pelvis is parallel to the seat. Check your head. Remember that the ears should be equidistant from the tops of the shoulders and the chin centered over the throat well.

When you lift the front spine, take care not to poke the lower front ribs forward, toward the chair back, or raise the shoulder yoke toward the ears. Maintain the normal curve of your lower back. Find a balance between the inward press of the sacrum and the downward lengthening of the tail. If you overdo the former, the lower back will arch too much; overdo the latter and the lower back will flatten or even bulge out.

When you move from reclining to sitting, not only will your body have to make an adjustment in its relationship with gravity, but so also will your breath. In reclining, once your body is established in Corpse alignment, you can pretty much forget about it and just fasten your consciousness on your breath. When you sit, though, you have to pay attention not only to your breath but to your physical alignment as well.

Aspirants report that their body is more defined when they sit. That's not surprising, since, as I mentioned earlier (in chapter 9), your normally-perceived physical boundaries tend to dissolve in a well-performed Corpse. But they add that their sitting breathing becomes shallower when compared to their reclining breathing.

This is an enormous source of despair and frustration for many students. All their hard work in developing their reclining breathing seems as if it's tossed out the window, and their practice is back to "Go." Be on the alert for this possibility and be prepared to spend some time—days, weeks, or months—acclimatizing yourself to your new position. Periodically return to reclining to reinforce your breathing memory, then try to re-create that same breath in Chair Seat.

Some students are reluctant to sit on a chair for yoga. One novice breather, who had studied asana for about a year, told me that sitting in a chair made her feel like a raw beginner again and self-conscious in a public class. I believe that everyone, regardless of their asana experience, should start their sitting pranayama practice in the Chair Seat. In the end how we look to ourselves and others in the sitting position is far less important than being steady and comfortable for the duration of our practice.

Transition from Chair Seat to Floor Sitting

How long should you practice pranayama in Chair Seat before you begin sitting in a traditional seat on the floor? (See chapter 16.) We've already asked a similar question in regard to the transition from reclining to Chair Seat. Again, the answer depends on your starting point, your commitment, and your karmic inheritance. Ask yourself two questions: Do I have a strong asana practice? And do I have a strong Chair Seat practice? In other words, am I preparing myself for the rigors of sitting with asana, and can I breathe comfortably with Conqueror and Against-the-Grain, the two foundation breaths (see chapters 18 and 19), for fifteen to twenty minutes? Expect to work with Chair Seat for around three months, including the time you spend transitioning into and out of the chair.

If your asana and reclining practices aren't that strong, delay practicing in a traditional floor seat until you can confidently answer yes to the above questions. Be aware that for some students the transition from the chair to the floor is a breeze, but for others it's more like a hurricane. Even though you can answer yes to the above questions, there's still no assurance that you're ripe for the floor. Again, don't despair if you run into obstacles.

When you feel you're just about ready to move from Chair Seat to floor sitting, sit on the floor for five to ten minutes near the end of your asana practice or end your reclining practice and precede Corpse with a few minutes in floor sitting. You could also sit on the floor, instead of that nice, big easy chair or couch, while you're watching TV or having an informal lunch at home, just to reinforce what you're practicing.

During this preliminary period, sit cross-legged on the floor, with your hands resting softly on your thighs, knees, or lap, eyes closed. Take a few minutes just to witness your floor-sitting behavior. It may not be very pretty, particularly if you're not accustomed to floor sitting, but try not to adjust yourself in any way; just sit and observe. What would you say now about the question Who is the sitter?

Then, during the last week or two of your Chair Seat practice, finish your asana practice and/or your pranayama practice with a few minutes in a traditional seat, witnessing the everyday breath.

Whether you're a beginning or an intermediate student, be sure to sit on a lift—either a bolster, a folded blanket, or a block—in whichever of these three seats you take. How high should the lift be? Use what you divined in the Chair Seat as a yardstick. Build up the height of your lift until you can sit comfortably on the fronts of your sitting bones with soft groins and a long front spine. You can gradually drop down as your work in asana opens your hips and groins and strengthens your back.

PLAYING AROUND: CHAIR SEAT

Don't forget to put into play what you learn in the Chair Seat as you go about your daily sitting business, at your desk, waiting at the bus stop, or just taking in the view from your favorite hillside or seashore spot.

When you sit at your desk, for example, sit forward near the front edge of the seat and try to avoid leaning against the back as much as you can. Ground the heads of your femurs and tailbone into the chair seat and lift the front spine through your crown. Lean forward over your desk from the hips, not by collapsing and shortening the front spine. Take periodic breaks from your sitting—rock the pelvis side to side, twist or lean right and left, do a back bend over the chair back.

LAST WORD

Proper sitting itself substantially contributes to quieting the fluctuations of citta and liberating the authentic breather. You can try this experiment on yourself. Sit on your chair and slump, doing your best depressed or fatigued person imitation. Roll onto the back of your sitting bones and let the spine, shoulders, and head curve forward. Take a few minutes to witness your body-mind and breath. Ask yourself: Who is the sitter? Who is the breather?

Then sit in your best Chair Seat. You can take a few minutes to witness your new situation, though I'd be surprised if you didn't feel the transformation almost immediately. Ask again: Who is the sitter? Who is the breather? You might write your answers and insights down in your journal.

CHAPTER 16

Traditional Seats

Holding his body steady with the three [that is, head,
    chest, neck] erect,
And causing the senses with the mind to enter into
    the heart,
A wise man with the Brahma-boat should cross over
All the fear-bringing streams.

Having repressed his breathings here in the body, and
    having his movements checked,
One should breathe through his nostrils with diminished
    breath.

—Shvetashvatara-Upanishad, in
The Thirteen Principal Upanishads,
translated by Robert Ernest Hume

GHERANDA AND SVATMARAMA together describe at least eight
floor seats that are suitable for pranayama. Traditionally the aspirant
sits on a flat surface, either the floor or a low platform called an
asana. His back is unsupported, though the lower back is sometimes
secured, and so supported, by a prop called a yoga cloth, a variation of which I'll describe in the "Easy Posture" section below, and
his legs are crossed in some fashion in front of the torso at the same
level as or slightly lower than the pelvis. This arrangement forms a
wide base of support, which opens and grounds the groins, lengthens the spine, and frees the diaphragm. Often the sitter's heels press
on sensitive areas of his body, such as the perineum or genitals, to
stimulate the vital energy and seal it in the torso.

The three seats I've chosen to work with in this guide are safe
and easy to perform without the supervision of a teacher. Easy posture (sukhasana) and Perfect posture (siddhasana) are familiar

cross-legged positions. Easy posture is probably best for beginning asana students, while Perfect posture, which requires more openness in the hips and groins, is suitable for intermediates. If you find these cross-legged positions difficult, then try the kneeling Hero posture (Svatmarama calls it bhadrasana, the Auspicious posture, which we'll discuss later in the chapter). If all three of these seats are difficult for you, then I recommend that you stay with the Chair Seat and look for a teacher who can give you some hands-on help.

A Detour Regarding Lotus Posture (Padmasana)

You may be wondering about the Lotus posture (padmasana), one of the most universally recognized of the yoga seats. If you've never sat in Lotus before, it's hard to appreciate just what a powerful seat it is and why it's so highly regarded and widely used for pranayama and meditation. Its unique leg-and-foot cross-lock creates an enormously steady and comfortable position, which naturally induces a meditative state.

But I'm not including this seat in this guide because, for most Westerners, Lotus is not only difficult to perform but potentially harmful as well. If you're practicing Lotus on your own, following instructions from a book or magazine, I strongly urge you to get instruction from an experienced teacher before you go any further. Unless you sufficiently prepare your hips and groins, and understand how to properly enter and leave the posture, Lotus can cause serious injury to your knees.

PRELIMINARY

Don't worry too much about your breathing when you first sit on the floor. Again, as with Chair Seat, accustom yourself physically to your new position before working with your breath. Call on your Witness, your best pranayama friend, to check the everyday breath. Who's the breather now? What happens to the breather when she flips herself upright in the gravity field? Record your observations in your journal.

If you're just beginning your sitting practice on the floor, you may not be quite ready to sit with an unsupported back. Since most of us habitually lean against a chair back when we sit, it's common for beginners' unsupported backs to start aching very quickly in yoga seats. If this is your situation, take the support of your yoga wall.

PRACTICE

For this practice you'll need your yoga wall and, depending on your preference of the wall-supported seats, either a rolled-up towel or a block. Position the sitting lift near or against your yoga wall. Settle down so that your sacrum and shoulder blades, but not the back of your head, contact the wall. To help support your lower back, put the rolled-up towel between it and the wall (see fig.16.1).

There's also a kind of halfway wall-supported position, which gets you mostly away from the wall but still provides some support. Position your sitting lift slightly away from the wall. Measure your distance from the wall so that you're sitting just a little closer than the long

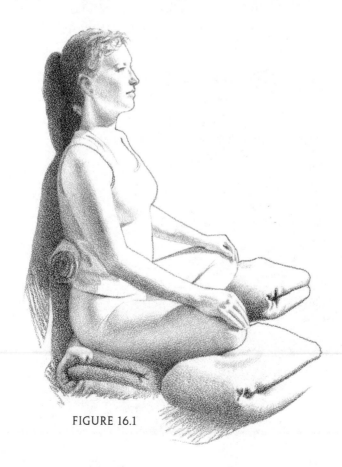

FIGURE 16.1

axis of your block, about eight inches on average. Wedge the block securely between your sacrum and the wall (see fig.16.2).

GOING FURTHER

I'll describe another way to support your back in the section on Perfect posture. Over time you'll want to strengthen your back with asanas, especially back bends, and consistent sitting practice and gradually move away from the wall.

Easy Posture (Sukhasana)

Sukha has an interesting etymology. Its antipode is duhkha (which we first ran across in chapter 2). The first syllable, *su*, means "good," "excellent," "beautiful," "easy," and the second, *kha*, is "the hole in the nave of a wheel through which the axle runs." Its original meaning, then, is "having a good axle hole," which no doubt was important for

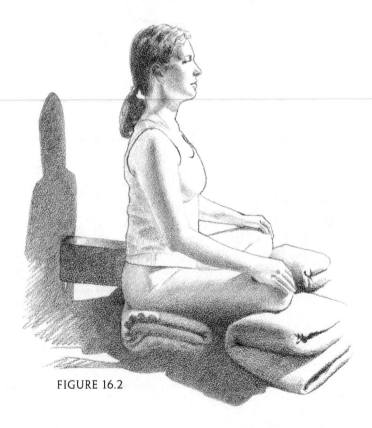

FIGURE 16.2

chariot wheels a few thousand years ago, before pneumatic tires, shock absorbers, and paved roads. *Sukha* generally means "pleasant," "agreeable," "gentle," "mild," "comfortable," "happy," "easy."

Gheranda calls this position Prosperous posture (svastikasana).

PRACTICE

The Easy posture is easy enough for most people, but not for everyone. If you're a beginning sitter with tight groins, get at least three blankets—or if you're sitting on a bolster, two blankets—and a couple of sandbags. If you want to try the variation I'll describe in "Going Further," then you'll also need a pair of straps.

Sit on the edge of a thickly folded blanket or bolster and cross your legs in front of you, each foot under the opposite thigh. Fold two blankets and put one under each of your outer thighs. Support the knees a little above where they would otherwise naturally fall. This blanket support is especially important if you want to use the sandbags, which you can lay across the very top of the inner thighs, parallel to the creases of the groins (see fig. 16.3).

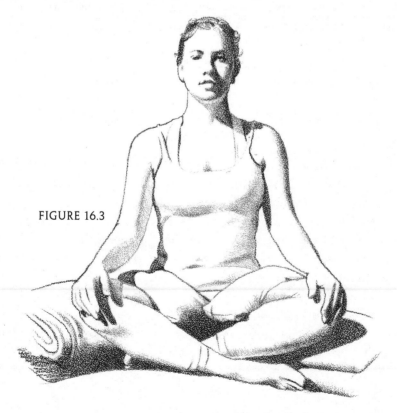

FIGURE 16.3

On Crossing the Legs

Sit down on the floor right now and, without thinking about it too much, cross your legs in the Easy posture. Which is the forward leg? Right or left? Being creatures of habit, we all tend to cross the legs in the same way every time we sit. It's important to remember, though, to alternate the cross of the legs from day to day to avoid, over time, unbalancing the hips.

Here's my strategy for remembering which way to cross the legs each day: on even-numbered days of the month, the right leg is the forward or higher leg, depending on the posture, while on odd-numbered days, it's the left leg. Be sure to apply this formula to the Perfect posture, too. I try not to worry that there are seven more odd-numbered days in a year than even.

HOW IT HELPS

Easy posture gets you ready for floor sitting in pranayama. Most of us can assume this position with relative ease, which gives us a feeling of confidence about what is, to many of us, a strange, new experience.

Caution. Never put the heavy bags on the inner thighs without supporting the outer thighs, or on the inner knees, even if the thighs are supported.

GOING FURTHER

Here's a variation of the yoga cloth (yoga-patta, mentioned in chapter 4) that will help you create a more stable and comfortable sitting position.

Buckle the two straps into large loops. Slip one loop over your torso and bring it down loosely over the outside of the left hip, just into the crease between the hip and thigh, and the cap of the right knee. Lift the knee an inch or so off the blanket, snug the loop over the hip and knee, then lower the knee back to its support. Repeat with the second loop and the right hip and left knee. When you're done, the two loops together will brace the back of your pelvis and cross in a kind of double X in front of you (see fig. 16.4).

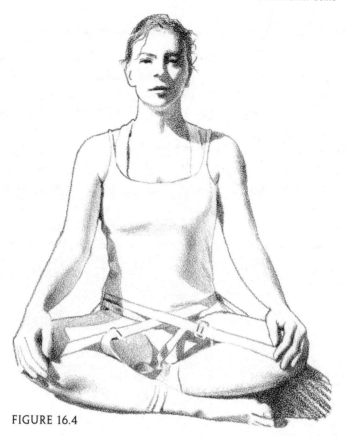

FIGURE 16.4

Now, as you continue to release the inner groins toward the floor, away from the bags, push each knee into its loop. Imagine that the two loops are gently pressing the sacrum evenly into the pelvis.

You can also use these yoga straps for the following seat (Perfect posture). Experiment with the sandbags and the straps until you're confident that you can re-create the movement of the groins and the sacrum and knees without them.

Perfect Posture (Siddhasana)

Siddha means "accomplished," "successful," "perfected," "endowed with supernatural faculties," "sacred." A siddha is someone who is accomplished at or perfected in yoga.

PRACTICE

In Perfect posture your knees will ideally drop a little closer to or fully onto the floor. You may need a blanket and, if you want to weigh down the groins as you did in Easy posture, two or more sandbags. If you want to try the variation I'll describe in "Going Further," then you'll also need a folding chair.

Sit on the edge of a thickly folded blanket with your legs crossed loosely in front of you. Draw the left heel close to, but not touching, the right groin. Slip the outer edge of the right foot in between the left thigh and calf, so that the right heel is near the left groin. Now pull both heels in to touch their opposite groins and slip the inner edge of the left foot in between the right thigh and calf (see fig. 16.5).

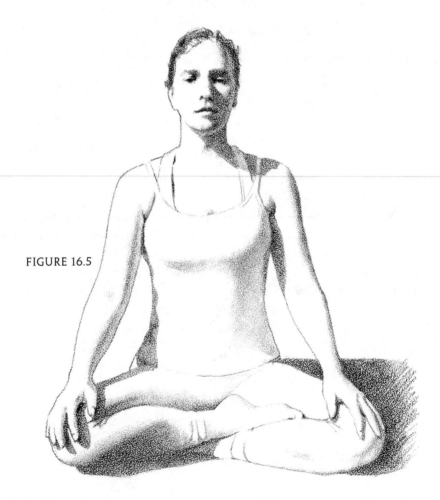

FIGURE 16.5

Put a folded blanket under your right knee if, like most beginning sitters, it doesn't easily rest on the floor. Lay the sandbags across the very top of the inner thighs, parallel to the creases of the groins.

HOW IT HELPS

The old guides value Perfect posture just as much as Lotus as a stable platform for sitting pranayama. "Just as moderate diet is the most important of the yamas, and non-violence of the niyamas, so the siddhas know that siddhasana is the most important of the asanas. Of all the eighty four asanas, siddhasana should always be practised. It purifies the 72,000 nadis."[1]

Physically Perfect posture stretches the ankles, groins, and hips; bathes the pelvic region with fresh blood; and spontaneously lengthens the front spine and so frees the diaphragm.

GOING FURTHER

Here's a version of the yoga table (yoga-pattaka). It will help you maintain the length of your spine and the lift of your upper torso during pranayama.

Fold two or three blankets lengthwise for your sitting support. My folded blankets measure about twelve-inches-by-twenty-four inches. Lay the blankets about twelve-inches-to-fifteen inches away from your yoga wall, with the long axis parallel to the wall. Now position the chair: brace the top edge of the chair back against the wall and set the feet of the front legs on the blankets, so that they touch an imaginary line that divides the blankets in half lengthwise.

Sit on the front half of the blankets, with your back torso, ideally in the area of the lower tips of the shoulder blades, pressing against the front edge of the chair seat (see fig. 16.6). Depending on your proportions relative to the dimensions of the chair, you may have to make one or two small adjustments:

- If there's not enough of the blankets projecting forward of the chair to provide a comfortable seat, move the blankets an inch or two farther from the wall.

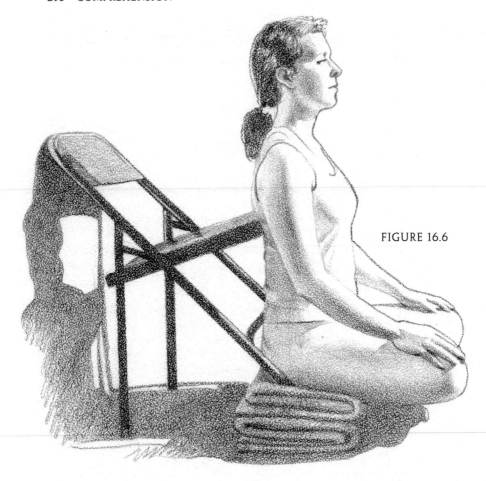

FIGURE 16.6

- If the edge of the chair seat contacts you too high on the back, place another folded blanket under your buttocks but not under the feet of the chair.

Hero Posture (Virasana)

We looked at Half Hero (ardha virasana) in chapter 14. The traditional version of the full Hero posture is often different than its modern counterpart. Gheranda instructs us, for example, to bring the left leg into Half Hero and the right into Half Lotus. Here, though, is the modern version of Hero.

PRACTICE

Not too many beginning sitters can sit in Hero with their buttocks on the floor. Get a block or two for a sitting support and, as usual, a sandbag or two to weigh down the groins. If you want to try the variation I'll describe below in "Going Further," you'll need a second block, or if you own only one block, you'll need to sit on something else, like a thick book.

Kneel on the floor with your knees together and your feet separated slightly wider than your hips. Point your feet straight back and spread the tops of the feet on the floor. Position the block between your feet with its long axis perpendicular to your inner ankles, so that when you sit, both of your sitting bones are well supported (see figs.16.7 a and b).

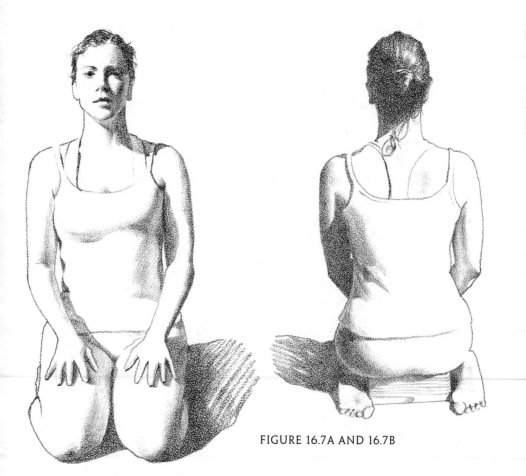

FIGURE 16.7A AND 16.7B

Press the web of each hand into the back of the same-side knee, thumb in, fingers out. As you sit back onto the block, turn the calves from the inside to the outside, sliding the thumbs out of the backs of the knees as the outer thighs contact the inner calves.

Keep the knees close together but position the inner heels a half inch or so away from the outer hips. Again, with your hands, pull the skin and flesh of the buttocks, just below the sitting bones, away from the back of the thighs and out toward the hips. Rest your hands, palms down, on your thighs.

Lay the heavy bag across the very top thighs to help release the groins. If you have two bags, lay one on each of the top thighs parallel to the crease of the groins. Be sure that your sitting bones are resting evenly on the block. If your knees slide apart, snug a strap around the thighs and shins or squeeze a thin book between your thighs.

Caution. Always approach Hero with caution. Pay particular attention to your knees, especially if you've had problems with them in the past. If one or both of your knees hurt, raise the height under your buttocks until the pain stops or wedge a thinly rolled dishtowel between the calf and thigh at the back of the knee. If you try these tricks and the pain doesn't stop, don't try to be a hero and tough it out—get out of the posture and seek the help of an experienced teacher.

If one or both of your ankles hurt, raise the height under your buttocks until the pain goes away or wedge a thinly rolled dishtowel underneath each ankle.

GOING FURTHER

To help the lift of your spine in Hero posture, position yourself a few inches from your yoga wall in Hero. Slide a block into the space between your sacrum and the wall, so that the block is firmly wedged in place and presses against the bone. Soften your belly and imagine that the bone is moving evenly into your pelvis (see fig. 16.2).

Common Problems in Floor Sitting

Most physical sitting problems involve some kind of discomfort in the feet, the knees, and the back. Often a simple self-adjustment is enough to solve the problem. Sometimes, though, if it persists, you'll need to consult with an experienced teacher.

My legs and feet fall asleep. If you're a beginning sitter, unaccustomed to sitting still on the floor in a cross-legged position, it's not unusual for your legs and feet to fall asleep after only a short while. It's a terrible feeling when your legs and feet start going numb and you wonder if you'll ever be able to run in a marathon again.

Short-term solutions:

- Sit on a higher support.
- Raise the knees from the floor onto a blanket support in Perfect posture or raise the height of the existing support in Easy posture.
- Change the cross of the legs at regular intervals—say, every few minutes.
- Cross the legs more loosely in Easy posture.
- Change your sitting position; for example, instead of Perfect posture, try Easy posture or sit on the chair.

Long-term solutions:

- Work on opening groins in your regular asana practice. Be sure not to tough it out if your feet fall asleep and start to tingle or, worse, go numb. Stretch your legs out and twist and shake them until the tingling goes away.
- Practice every day for a set length of time—say, five to ten minutes at first. When you start to feel comfortable with this time, then gradually extend the time of your practice a minute or so a week until you can sit comfortably for fifteen to twenty minutes. With regular practice you'll be surprised at how quickly you can adapt to the sitting position.

My back hurts. Most everyday chairs have a back, and we chair sitters love to lean against this back when we sit. Over time, of course, we get addicted to this support, and when we're asked to sit without it, we feel lost. Unsupported, we tend to slump forward, humping our back, which is, to a yoga teacher, like waving the proverbial red cape in front of a bull. Most teachers will sneak up behind you and poke you somewhere on the back torso, encouraging you to, as your mother might have reminded you when you were a child, "sit up straight." I don't really want you to do that, because we don't actually want a straight spine, just a long one that preserves its natural curves. Unused to holding the spine long with only the muscles of the spine, the beginning sitter usually lasts only a minute or so before the slump returns. On an unprepared back, the demands of maintaining a long spine inevitably lead to an aching back.

Short-term solutions:

- Sit on a higher support.
- Sit against a support like your yoga wall or chair.
- Take regular stretch breaks every five minutes or so. You can twist from side to side, lean forward, bend backward, and so forth.

Long-term solutions:

- Again, as with sleeping legs and feet, the best long-term solution is regular practice. Of course, the back is uncomfortable at first, but given time, it begins to learn how to support itself comfortably. Remember, too, in your everyday sitting, to rely as little as you can on your chair's back support. Sit forward on the seat, away from the chair back, or use only a lumbar roll made with a firmly rolled-up towel to support your lower back.
- Recognize, though, that sometimes an aching back is due to some chronic condition, such as scoliosis, which is a lateral curvature of the spine. For a challenging situation like this, you'll need the assistance of an experienced teacher.

I can't stop fidgeting. Judging by the comments in aspirants' journals, it's a chore for many sitters to sit still for more than a few minutes. Sometimes the fidgeting is instigated by physical discomfort, but many times it's all in your head—those fluctuations again—which unfortunately gets expressed in your body as a serious case of the heebie-jeebies.

Short-term solutions:

- Start your sitting practice with just a few minutes a day and gradually, over the weeks and months of your sitting career, increase your sitting time.

- First spend a few minutes in Corpse before you sit for pranayama. See if you can use Corpse to quiet the vrittis, then bring that quality of Corpse-mind into your sitting position.

- When you sit, wrap your head, though not your eyes, firmly with an elastic bandage (see chapter 10 for details).

- If you have sandbags or barbell weights, put everything on the heads of your thighbones. I've had as much as one hundred pounds sitting on my thighs. This helps to soften the groins and, in turn, the brain. Remember, though, if your knees are off the floor, support them on blocks or thickly folded blankets.

Long-term solutions:

- Practice sitting daily for gradually increasing increments of time. For example, start your sitting practice with a reasonably short stay—say, three minutes. Practice at this time until you can sit fairly steadily.

- Then increase your sitting stay by, say, ten or fifteen seconds and practice at this time until you can sit without fidgeting.

- Proceed in this fashion, aiming for an attainable short-term sitting goal, maybe five minutes. Then go celebrate, come back, and aim for ten minutes using the same procedure. After a few years you'll be sitting pretty.

As I've mentioned, fidgeting is frequently a reaction to our unbridled fluctuations. As with the charioteer and his horses, we need to bring these fluctuations under our control, though not through force and coercion. Remember that the fluctuations are nothing more than surface perturbations on the vast sea of consciousness. With the help of your Witness, learn to look beneath the superficial unrest at the eternal stillness in the heart of each of us.

LAST WORD

Now that you've worked with the asanas and know something about the reclining and sitting positions, everything's in place for the last leg of our journey. We'll next work with the two foundation breaths of the practice and learn a few supporting techniques that will help carry us to our final destination.

PART FOUR

Completion

CHAPTER 17

Tools
Upaya

If you observe your natural inclinations, there is a certain point where the whole yoga practice will come to you. We are having to learn it by prescription because we are not sensitive to whatever is natural in us.

—Usharbudh Arya, *Philosophy of Hatha Yoga*

EVERY TRAVELER uses tools, such as backpacks and maps, to get around from place to place. Travelers to the country of the Self also have tools—called *upaya*, or "means"—practical techniques that are part of every formal training, which help them along on the path of liberation.

Traditionally these tools are passed on to the aspirant by her teacher. As a beginner, the tools you need are fairly simple, but as you get farther into the country of the Self, they get more powerful and complex. At first you'll handle your tools rather clumsily, but over time, as you repeatedly use them, you'll get more adept. It's almost as if they become a part of you.

In preparation for the Conqueror and Against-the-Grain breaths (which we'll work with in the next two chapters), we'll learn to handle five tools in this chapter: hymn, or mantra; hand seals; an exercise I call nasal balance; Skull Brightener (kapalabhati); and ratio breathing. In general these tools help to quiet the body-mind and stimulate and regulate the movement of the breath. They reinforce the Witness and so gather awareness toward the breath and the self and help to cultivate self-understanding.

Hymn (Mantra)

A mantra is literally a "prayer" or "hymn," though it bears little resemblance to our Western ways of praying or singing hymns. The yogis say that the word derives from the first syllable of manana, which means "thinking," "reflection," "meditation," and the suffix tra, which suggests an instrument. A mantra, then, is an instrument of thought or meditation, a word of power, a mystic sound or formula, a call or channel to the divine. It may consist of a single syllable, called a seed, or bija; a string of syllables; a word; or an entire sentence. Some mantras have a literal meaning, while others seem to be merely sounds. But these sounds can switch off the fluctuations of citta. They relay hidden messages about extraordinary states of consciousness and self-liberation that couldn't otherwise be expressed in everyday rational language.

For a mantra to be truly effective, tradition says it must be planted in your heart by a self-realized teacher, properly pronounced with due attention to its secret meaning, never revealed to anyone else, and meditated on silently rather than chanted aloud.

Mantras traditionally have three purposes: They protect from disease, evil spirits, and spells and gain the favor of a particular god. They confer magical powers, called siddhis. And they invoke and intensify our identity with the Highest Reality.

Unspoken Hymn (Ajapa-mantra)

There is a pair of mantras that are effortlessly and ceaselessly recited by every creature, breath after breath, throughout its life. They are the means by which the universe itself initiates us into the mysteries of breathing. Together they're called the unspoken mantra (ajapa-mantra). According to yoga tradition, each in-breath and out-breath makes a distinct sound. Listen carefully, we're told, and you'll hear in the exhalation an aspirate HA and in the inhalation a sibilant SA, though in some old guidebooks these sounds are reversed. These two syllables are arranged into two different mantras. One is HAMSA, which in Sanskrit is a migratory bird, usually pictured as a swan or wild goose. Heinrich Zimmer explains that this bird is an "animal mask"[1] of both the universal creative impulse and the self-realized saint. It "symbolizes the divine essence, which, though embodied in, and abiding with, the individual, yet remains forever free from, and unconcerned with, the events of individual life."[2]

The second form of the mantra reverses the two syllables—SAHAM, sometimes spelled SOHAM. SA connotes "that," the Great Self (parama-atman) or brahman. HA connotes "I," the living self (jiva-atman), the self that lives in each of us. In its two forms the unspoken mantra acknowledges and affirms that "I am the divine life-principle revealed in the melody of the breath."[3]

PRACTICE

The sound of ajapa-mantra is created by slightly contracting and then breathing through the space between your vocal cords, called the glottis, which acts like a valve to control the movement of air. The vocal cords are in your larynx, which is marked by that little bump on the front of your throat we popularly call the Adam's apple.

Let's start with the HA sound. Gently pinch the front of your throat, on either side of your larynx, with the thumb and forefinger of one hand. Inhale through your nose, then open and form your lips into an O shape and exhale through your mouth. Pass the out-breath over the back of your throat, just behind the larynx, and vocalize a long, slow HA. It should sound as if you were fogging a mirror with your breath or blowing warm air into your palms on a cold day. You'll notice that, in order for you to make the sound itself, the glottis naturally narrows. Try this a few times, until you can feel the vocal cords contracting and hear the HA clearly.

Next, close your mouth and inhale through your nose. Continue to gently pinch the front of your throat. Narrow your glottis and exhale with a HA over the back of the throat again but this time through your nose. A fair number of students say they don't really hear the HA, but that's OK. Just listen for the sound of the breath, whatever sound it seems to make to you.

Now empty as much air as you can from your lungs by contracting your abdominal muscles and exhaling through your nose. Then pinch your throat the same way as before and lightly constrict your glottis. Inhale through your nose and, as you did with HA, pass the breath over the back of your throat with a long, slow SA. Again, there are reports from the field that SA is nowhere to be found, but again, don't worry. It's enough at first to make a sound—any sound—on the exhales and inhales. The HAS and SAS will come to you with practice.

For me the HA is created a little lower in the throat, behind the larynx, while the SA is made higher, at the back of the soft palate. The texture of the two syllables should be very smooth from the beginning of either the inhale or the exhale until its end. Inhale the SA up the front of your spine; exhale the HA down the back.

HOW IT HELPS

The ajapa-mantra naturally slows the time of your breath and so affects texture, space, and rest. The sound of the mantra also helps to interiorize consciousness and soothe its fluctuations.

Caution. Be careful not to overly contract the glottis—the amplified sounds require a light touch, not a death grip. And don't force the sound of the mantra if you can't hear it right away. Some students complain that the mantra causes throat tension and soreness. If this is the case with you, then do two or three mantraless cycles of breath between each mantra cycle.

PLAYING AROUND: SONG OF THE DIVINE

Be sure to tune in to this mantra throughout your day. Set your digital watch, if you can, to beep on the hour as a reminder to check in regularly with this song of the divine, the source, sustenance, and goal of our lives.

Hand Seals (Hasta-mudra)

Mudra is literally defined as a "seal," in the sense of any instrument used for sealing or stamping something else. According to the tenth-century sage Abhinavagupta, there are four different types of mudra, which are made by the whole body, by the hands, by speech (or the mouth or tongue), and in consciousness only.

Like most words in the yoga lexicon, mudra has both a literal meaning and esoteric interpretations. In some old guides a mudra is said to be that which gives (ra) joy or pleasure (muda) to the gods. Others explain a mudra as that which dissolves or melts spiritual bondage (mu) or that which seals (mudranat) the entire universe in a state of enlightenment.

As a bodily position, a mudra is intended to seal the life force in the body, where it may be used for pranayama and meditation. When it's created only with the hands, a mudra helps us to realize certain states of consciousness by mimicking ritual or symbolic gestures. The knowledge of mudra is supposed to grant magical or divine powers, produce stability and firmness in the body-mind by giving control over nerves and muscles, cure diseases, purify the nadis, and ultimately assist in the awakening of kundalini. I'll describe three basic seals below.

PRELIMINARY

Stretch your hands wide, splaying the fingers out from the center of the palms like the spokes of a wheel. Then shake them a few times.

PRACTICE

Probably the best-known hand seal is the Wisdom Seal (jnana-mudra). Touch the tip of your index finger to the tip of your thumb, forming a circle with these two fingers. Then extend the remaining fingers away from your palm.

As I mentioned above, seals have ritual or symbolic import. In the Wisdom Seal, the thumb represents the Great Self (parama-atman); the index finger, the embodied self (jiva-atman); the other three fingers, the three strands or qualities (guna)—energy (rajas), inertia (tamas), and luminosity or beingness (sattva)—that compose the material world. The gesture symbolizes the union of the individual and divine selves, resulting in the transcendence of the mundane world.

A variation of the Wisdom Seal is called the Awareness Seal (cin-mudra), in which the tip of the index finger is brought to the root of the thumb.

You can perform these two seals with the palms either up or down. Generally speaking, palms down helps calm the brain and softens the shoulders and is most appropriate for beginning students; palms up opens the heart and stimulates the brain and is more suitable for experienced students.

One of the simplest seals is called Meditation Seal (dhyana-mudra) or sometimes Fierce Seal (bhairava-mudra). Here just lay your hands in your lap, with the back of the right hand resting in the palm of the left and the tips of your thumbs lightly touching. In some descriptions of this seal, the thumb tips aren't touching; instead, the thumbs are stacked, passively, one on top of the other. The feminine version of this seal (called bhairavi-mudra; note the feminine "i" ending here as opposed to the masculine "a" ending in the other spelling) reverses the position of the hands.

The left and right hands are said to stand for the comfort and tawny channels, respectively (ida-nadi and pingala-nadi; see the "Nasal Balance" section below), the contact of the hands, then the union of the two in the central channel (sushumna-nadi), the path to liberation.

HOW IT HELPS

There are a great number of hand seals applied to pranayama and meditation for many different reasons. In this guide we'll use a hand seal simply as another tool for steadying consciousness—as with fidgeting or agitation in the body or the eyes, nervous fingers and hands are said to cause fluctuations in consciousness.

Be aware, though, that the mudras are ultimately designed to seal life energy in the body. For example, according to some authorities, the contact of the thumb and index finger in the Wisdom and Awareness Seals creates a circuit or loop. This reverses the wasteful outward flow of energy through the fingertips and seals it in the body, where it can be used to cultivate and refine consciousness for breathing and meditation.

Nasal Balance

The yogis have known for a long time—and now modern science is confirming—that the flow of air through our nostrils is rarely ever equal. Usually one of the nostrils is partially or completely blocked. This nostril dominance, as it's sometimes called, alternates back and forth between the two throughout the day. Each cycle lasts somewhere between one and two hours.

This might not seem like a big deal. But the yogis have observed that this alternation of nostril dominance is associated with significant shifts in consciousness. This has again been corroborated by modern science—always the arbiter of truth in our Western culture. Left-nostril dominance, which is connected to the right brain hemisphere, is associated with the ida-nadi, and its nature is thought to be feminine and peaceful. Right-nostril dominance, on the other hand, is connected to the left hemisphere, associated with the pingala-nadi and everything masculine and aggressive.

Obviously, then, certain activities are more suitable to one or the other dominant nostril. If I'm breathing through my right nostril, for example, I want to be out there conquering worlds and climbing large mountains—or at least washing my car. But if I'm breathing through my left nostril, then I want to be doing something more sedentary, like playing my guitar—early Bob Dylan only—or reading a good novel. Of course, if I'm cornered into doing something active and my left nostril is dominant, then I either have to wait until the shift happens on its own or find a way to quickly coax it myself.

Leave it to the yogis to figure this latter technique out, but not because of any mundane reasons. They're actually looking not to shift their nasal dominance from one side to the other—although they might want to do this if, for example, they need right dominance for an especially vigorous asana session—but to balance the flow of breath in both nostrils.

Remember that balance (samatva) is a key word in the yoga lexicon; in fact, you could accurately render yoga itself into English as "balance." Equalizing the flow of breath in the two nostrils is said to quiet the fluctuations and is considered to be an important preparation for both pranayama and meditation.

Traditionally the yogis use a short staff (danda), shaped something like a crutch, to alter nostril dominance. They squeeze the head of this staff in the armpit on the side of the nondominant nostril to open it up. You have to wonder how anybody ever managed to figure this out. There's also an asana, favored by some practitioners, called the Yoga Staff posture (yoga-dandasana), in which the sole of your foot is inserted into your armpit (if you can't puzzle out what this might look like, then see the remarkable photo in *Light on Yoga*).

You'll notice that I didn't include one of these staffs in the props list (chapter 4) or the foot-in-the-armpit posture in the asana list (chapter 14). That's because there's something we all have that's a lot closer to hand, so to speak.

PRACTICE

The props you'll need for this exercise are one hand, balled into a fist, or an old tennis ball. Sit comfortably. Press your right index finger against the right wing of your nose and completely block the nostril. Take a few breaths through your left nostril to determine how the breath is flowing: is it relatively easy, or does the nostril feel a little stuffy? Then block the left nostril and breathe only through the right. What about now? Which nostril would you say is the more open or dominant?

Fist the hand of the dominant-nostril side and wedge it into the nondominant-nostril armpit. Squeeze the fist between your arm and side chest for a few minutes and again pay attention to the flow of breath in the targeted nostril.

HOW IT HELPS

The breathing balance between the right and left nostrils, writes Swami Saraswati, induces a "state of harmony and balance throughout the entire central nervous system, and the systems governing respiratory, circulatory, digestive and excretory functions." Moreover, he continues, the frontal lobes of the cerebrum are freed to work to their fullest potential, which leads to genius, intuition, and creativity.[4]

GOING FURTHER

Alternatively you could squeeze a tennis ball in the armpit or lie on your side with the dominant nostril down.

Skull Brightener (Kapalabhati)

Kapalabhati means "skull brightener" or "skull cleaner," from kapala, "skull," and bhati, "to make shine" or "to clean" (but also "perception" and "knowledge"). It's considered a milder form of, and a preparation for, its more powerful relative, with the somewhat formidable name of Bellows (bhastrika). Some guides list Skull Brightener as a pranayama, while others deem it a purification exercise. We'll use Skull Brightener as a preparation for pranayama proper.

In everyday breathing the inhalation is the active phase of the breath, since it requires the contraction of the main breathing muscle, the diaphragm. Conversely the exhalation is predominantly passive, generated as it is by the release of the diaphragm, though, of course, there are other muscles that contract to help push air out of the lungs. Also, the time of everyday inhalation is usually shorter than that of exhalation. With Skull Brightener these attributes of the two phases are reversed. Skull Brightener's exhalation is very fast, accomplished with a quick contraction of the lower belly muscles, which pushes the viscera up against the diaphragm. When this contraction is released, the viscera drop, pulling the diaphragm down and sucking air into the lungs.

In the following sections, you'll find two versions of Skull Brightener. The first is the milder of the two, performed while reclining with just the lightest touch of the fingertips on your lower belly as a tactile aid. The second version, then, is the more vigorous, done in a sitting position, with a slight alteration in the traditional technique. In most guides the exhale is accomplished with the unassisted contraction of the lower belly. In order to do that reasonably well, you have to train your belly muscles over a very long time. Here, though, we'll use our hands to assist with the belly pump. All breathing in Skull Brightener should be done through your nose.

PRACTICE: RECLINING SKULL BRIGHTENER

Using whatever props you use for reclining pranayama, lie on your support and lay your fingertips lightly on your lower belly. Breathe as you normally do into your lower belly and for a few minutes watch the rise and fall of the fingertips. Notice in particular how the lower belly firms during your exhales, helping to push the air out of your lungs.

To begin, take a moderate inhale and quickly contract your lower belly, pushing the air out of your lungs and through your nose with a sharp whoosh. Then just as quickly let go of the contraction and allow the air to be passively sucked back into your lungs. Try that a few times, separating each whooshing breath with a few everyday breaths.

Of course, you have to do this more than once to get the full effect of this exercise. As a beginning rule of thumb, exhale once every two or three seconds, for about ten to twelve times in the first round. Then wait thirty seconds to a minute with everyday breathing to see how things are going. Some students feel exhilarated, others faint. Ask yourself, Is one round enough, at least for the time being, or is another round possible? Perform from one to three rounds of ten to twelve breaths each, separating rounds one and two with thirty seconds to a minute of everyday breathing.

Spend a few weeks getting acquainted with reclining Skull Brightener at this relatively low level of work. Once you're sure you can handle this practice, slowly increase the speed of the exhalations and the number of exhalations per round. Use your best judgment about how rapidly to progress and when to switch your practice to the sitting version.

PRACTICE: SITTING SKULL BRIGHTENER

Get whatever props you need to make yourself comfortable in your favorite sitting position, whether in Chair Seat or on the floor. Cup the back of one hand in the palm of the other and make a light fist. Bring the pinky sides of the fist against your lower belly, just above the pubis. For a few minutes gently knead or churn your belly, pressing the fist in toward the spine and up toward the diaphragm. Imagine that you're first lifting the weight or mass of your belly, then release it and allow it to sink down again.

Notice what happens as you lift and release the weight of your belly. During the lift there's a gentle tug on the perineum, which hollows it slightly upward into the pelvis, and the pressure on the bottom of the diaphragm encourages a soft exhale. Release the weight and it reflexively sucks air into the lungs.

To begin, take a moderate inhale and then quickly press your hands diagonally up and into the belly, pushing the air out of your lungs and through your nose with a sharp *whoosh*. Then just as quickly let go of the lifted belly and watch how it rebounds, sucking air back into the lungs without any effort. Does your skull seem any brighter?

Of course, as with the reclining version, you have to do this more than once to get the full benefit of this exercise. Use the same beginning rule of thumb for sitting as for reclining: exhale once every two or three seconds, for about ten to twelve times in the first round. Then wait thirty seconds to a minute with everyday breathing to see how things are going. Are you exhilarated or about to keel over? Is one round enough, at least for the time being, or is another round possible? Perform from one to three rounds of ten to twelve breaths each, separating rounds one and two with thirty seconds to a minute of everyday breathing.

As before, take some time operating at this low level and, once you're comfortable, slowly increase the speed of the exhalations and the number of exhalations per round. Respect the lions, elephants, and tigers, just because you're working without the net of experienced supervision. Some guides note that it's possible to do 120 breaths in one minute, but this is surely the performance of a professional breather on a closed track. Aim for about three rounds of 50 breaths each over the next six months to a year.

HOW IT HELPS

According to traditional and modern guides, Skull Brightener has many benefits. It cleanses the sinuses, respiratory passages, and lungs and keeps the spongy tissue of the lungs supple. It saturates the blood with oxygen and stimulates cell breathing, which ensures good metabolic activity; improves the venous blood circulation by turning the diaphragm into a powerful pump; and irrigates, purifies, and invigorates the brain, pituitary, and pineal glands with oxygenated blood. It strengthens, massages, and tones abdominal muscles and organs, including the diaphragm and liver, and improves digestion.

I like Skull Brightener because it soothes my brain and gets me in the mood for pranayama. One old guide claims that it stimulates the energy centers at the solar plexus (manipura-chakra) and the so-called third eye, or ajna-chakra, at the middle of the forehead.

Incidentally, the Skull Brightener described here is technically known as air process (vatakrama). There are two related processes. One is called the inversion process (vyutkrama), in which you sniff salt water through your nose and spit it out your mouth, which is said to cure diseases of phlegm. Its opposite is the cooling process (shitkrama), in which you push a mouthful of salt water out through your nose, which is said to make you as beautiful as Kama, the Hindu Cupid—though presumably not at the same time the water is dribbling out of your nostrils.

Caution. Traditionally the yogis monitor five elements of Skull Brightener:

1. The vigor of the exhale, which is more important than speed. If you become dizzy, stop the practice and sit quietly for a while, breathing normally. When you start again, breathe with more awareness and less force. Remember to push the breath out with the lower belly only, keeping the upper belly, diaphragm, throat, face, and nostrils soft.

2. The speed of the breaths, which should increase slowly over time. Remember that the inhale should feel spontaneous, not forced, and that the exhale shouldn't make you breathless.

3. The number of breaths to a single round.

4. The number of rounds to a sitting.

5. The total number of sittings in one day, assuming that you practice pranayama more than once a day. In the old days the yogis practiced four times a day, every six hours—at dawn, noon, sunset, and midnight; think about this every time you complain about your once-a-day fifteen-minute session.

Ratio Breathing (Vritti Pranayama)

In general, ratio breathing is called vritti pranayama. We've run across the word vritti before, as the fluctuations of our consciousness. But in the context of pranayama practice, the word indicates a particular course of action, which is the purposeful regulated ratio of the times of the four phases of breathing.

There are two basic categories of ratios in pranayama, which are called equal ratio (sama-vritti) and unequal ratio (vishama-vritti). You can begin your practice of vritti pranayama in the reclining position, which is how I'll set you up in the practices that follow, and then continue on to move to a sitting practice. Be sure to gain some proficiency with equal ratio breathing before you take on unequal ratio, both when reclining and then again when sitting. Give yourself about two weeks to do this in each position. Like all of my recommmendations, though, this is only a minimum guideline, and how long you stay with equal ratio breathing depends on your response to this tool. Some students feel at ease right away and roll along merrily to unequal ratio in the minimum time. Others find equal ratio a challenge and stay with it for longer, sometimes much longer.

Over the centuries aspirants have experimented with different ratios and developed various ways to measure their time. In this guide we'll simply count silently to ourselves "one-om, two-om, three-om," and so on.

Equal Ratio (Sama-vritti)

Sama means "even," "smooth," "flat," "equal," "same." This Sanskrit word is the etymological parent of the English word same. In equal ratio, as the name suggests, the times of the inhalations and exhalations are the same. So, for example, if you inhale for four counts, you would also exhale for four counts. Equal ratio breathing is thought to induce a more equal or balanced state of consciousness.

PRACTICE

Taking whatever props you need for your reclining position, lie on your support and establish and count your most comfortable slow-breathing times. In this example we'll say that you've counted your inhalation time to six counts and your exhalation to eight. There are two ways to set up an equal ratio. The first is to adjust the longer breath to match the shorter. In our example decrease your exhale to equal the inhale, so that both equal six counts. Or add the two numbers together, then divide by two. In our example, six plus eight equals fourteen, and fourteen divided by two equals seven. If your two counts add up to an odd number, decrease the total by one before you divide. Then increase your inhalations and decrease your exhalations by one count each, so both equal seven counts.

For the purpose of illustration, let's look at the first method of equalizing the breaths. You'll be inhaling and exhaling to a count of six. It should be fairly easy for you to match six on your inhalation, since it's already your established comfortable count. But the exhalation may be a bit tricky at first. You might find yourself hurrying to get all the breath out by the six count, or you might reach six and still have another count or so of breath left over in your lungs. Keep at it. With practice and patience, there's no doubt you'll find the proper speed of exhale.

Once you're satisfied with this first count, which may take a few days or even longer, tack on another count and, to continue with our illustration, inhale and exhale to seven. Proceed in this fashion, accustoming yourself to a specific ratio for a few days and then adding one count to stretch the limits of your count, until you find a number that seems both stimulating and fulfilling.

Caution. Some students report that counting the breaths seems forced, that it distracts them from attending to the natural rhythm of the breath. "How can I count and observe my breath at the same time?" one student commented in her journal. Never force yourself in using any of these tools. If counting is a problem, just estimate the time of the inhalations and exhalations. You should be comfortable with equal ratio breathing before moving on to unequal ratio (below) and retention (chapter 20).

Unequal Ratio (Vishama-vritti)

Vishama means just the opposite of sama—"uneven," "irregular," "dissimilar," "odd." In unequal ratio pranayama, the times of inhalations and exhalations are different. Many ratios are possible, of course, but the one most favored in the old yoga guides is one count of inhalation to every two counts of exhalation—in other words, your exhalation is twice as long as your inhalation. This ratio is said to pacify the brain and nervous system and promote a meditative state of consciousness.

I've learned to create the unequal ratio—surprise!—as if I were taming lions, elephants, and tigers. I first match the exhale and inhale counts in equal ratio breathing, then slowly build up the exhale count until it doubles the inhale.

PRACTICE

Lie on your support and establish and count your most comfortable slow-breathing times. As in the equal ratio example, we'll say that this inhalation time is six. Now choose a number that is lower than this count. Let's be an archconservative—just for the purposes of this illustration, of course—and take three.

Establish equal ratio breathing for the inhalations and exhalations at three. You'll find there will be lots of room left in your lungs at the end of the inhalation, which is fine. Breathe to this reduced equal ratio for a few minutes, then increase the exhale by one count, so that the next counts will be three for the inhalation and four for the exhalation. Stay with these new counts for a few minutes more. Watch your breath and your reaction to it closely. Add the next count to the exhale only if you feel comfortable with four—and if you don't, stay with this count until you do. Then add one count more to the exhalation and inhale for three and exhale for five. Again, after a few minutes check your breath and, again, advance the exhale count only if you're content with five—and if you're not, stay where you are until you are. Finally, add that last count to the exhale to round out the classic one-to-two ratio.

Once you're satisfied with your first unequal ratio, which may take a few days or even longer, then add a count to your inhalation and (to continue with our illustration) increase it to four. Now inhale to four but continue to exhale to six for a few minutes. Then add one count to the exhalation, breathe for a few minutes, and if all is well, finally extend your exhalation out to eight. This is the pattern to follow to develop your unequal ratio breathing. When you've mastered a particular ratio, add one count to the inhale, gradually increase the exhale to double the inhale, then again up the ante on the inhalation by one, and so on and so forth, until you again reach a limit that is both stimulating and fulfilling.

HOW IT HELPS

The time of everyday breathing is unrhythmic or irregular. Sometimes our inhales are longer than the exhales, sometimes it's the other way round, and sometimes everything just comes to a dead stop and we hold our breath. As I've mentioned, yoga teaches that this inharmonious breathing is an outward show of the typically inharmonious state of our everyday consciousness. In pranayama the aspirant tries to steady and harmonize her consciousness, often as a prelude to meditation, by fixing a ratio between the times of the inhales and the times of the exhales. Sama-vritti, as its name suggests, is said to create a quality of "sameness" or balance in the flow of consciousness. Vishama-vritti, which lengthens the exhale, further calms the fluctuations.

Caution. Be sure to master the active phases of the breath, the inhales and exhales, in ratio breathing before you add the two phases of breathing pauses to the equation.

Don't struggle to reach the one-to-two ratio. It's perfectly acceptable to stop somewhere short of doubling the time of the exhalation. For example, you could inhale for four and exhale for seven and work at that level for a while until you feel comfortable enough to add the final count.

PLAYING AROUND: RATIOS

As you proceed with your practice, it might be interesting to investigate a variety of ratios. For example, you could lengthen the exhale count $2\frac{1}{2}$ or three times the inhale count or reverse the classic one-to-two ratio and take two counts of inhalation for every one count of exhalation.

LAST WORD

Though we use mantra, ratio breathing, and Skull Brightener in formal training, the foundation of pranayama is always the bare witnessing of the authentic breath. Find this breath first before you pick up the tools in this chapter. And while world travelers will always need their tools to help them get around, as travelers in the country of the Self, we'll eventually leave them behind. As the journey of the authentic breath nears completion in kevala-kumbhaka, you'll abandon your breathing tools by the side of the road.

CHAPTER 18

Conqueror's Breath
Ujjayi Pranayama

Close the mouth, draw in the external air by both nostrils,
and pull up the internal air from the lungs and throat;
retain them in the mouth. . . . Let a man perform Ujjayi
to destroy decay and death.

—Gheranda on ujjayi pranayama,
Gheranda-Samhita, translated by
Rai Bahadur Srisa Chandra Vasu

THERE ARE MORE than a dozen different pranayamas. Svatmarama
and Gheranda each list eight, though not the same eight, while B. K. S.
Iyengar, in his *Light on Pranayama*, lists fourteen. But we'll only
work with two breaths in this guide, Conqueror (ujjayi) and Against-
the-Grain (viloma). It's my feeling that, for the first year or so of
practice, it's more than enough work to establish witnessing consciousness, map our body and the qualities of everyday breath, refine
these qualities, and then learn a couple of foundation pranayamas
with simple supporting tools.

Ujjayi means "to win," "to conquer," "to acquire by conquest," "to
be victorious." The name is partly suggested, it seems, by the way
the aspirant swells her chest out like a proud conqueror, in order to
maximize the capacity of her lungs. Hidden in this word is the little prefix *ud*, which means "up," in the sense of superiority in place,
rank, or power. This also suggests that ujjayi is a superior or powerful technique for liberation, a tool by which the yogis can conquer
the forces of ignorance and bondage.

Four Stages of Daily Practice

In general, each of your Conqueror and Against-the-Grain practice sessions will have four stages. These stages apply whether you're in the reclining or sitting position. How long you spend in the reclining position before shifting to sitting depends a lot on you. According to the practice outline schedule in appendix 1, the minimum amount of time you can expect to recline before sitting upright is about six months.

If you've done your homework with unusual breathing (chapter 12), then nothing in this chapter and the one that follows on Against-the-Grain will seem very unusual to you. Conqueror is simply the purposeful or conscious application of the simple lessons learned from slow, stop-and-wait, and spot breathing (we'll get to zigzag in the next chapter). You might say that Conqueror is the fulfillment or completion of those exercises. Take spot breathing, for example; in Conqueror, instead of dividing the torso into various spots, the torso as a whole becomes the spot, as you attempt to full-fill the entire inner space.

PRELIMINARY

Be certain you have all your props handy before you start your practice. It can be very frustrating to lie down, for example, and then realize you left your watch or eye bag in another room.

Remember to prepare yourself mentally for your practice. Acknowledge and affirm your commitment to your work and its ultimate goal of self-fulfillment.

Determine your nostril dominance. Use the squeezed-fist technique to open, as much as possible, the nondominant nostril. Then perform Skull Brightener to your capacity. Once you've finished all this, rest your hands in your favorite hand seal.

Stage 1

Whether reclining or sitting, balance yourself physically first. Remember that the measuring stick for balance is your midline, and in neutral positions like reclining or sitting, the midline follows the front of your spine, what I've called the heart axis.

Then take a couple of minutes to check in with your everyday breath. Don't do anything yet; just witness and allow your breath to be itself, even with all its flaws and imperfections. Clarify, but don't alter, its time, texture, and space. Ask yourself the question Who is the breather? Just as you're not trying to breathe, but simply allowing yourself to be breathed, don't try to answer this question. Allow the question to be answered.

Witnessing in this way day after day requires you to walk a kind of breathing tightrope. Obviously, over the weeks of your practice, you'll get more and more familiar with your breathing identity. A stranger at first, it will grow to be an old friend after a while. The danger is in becoming too familiar and forgetting that your breathing identity is incrementally changing as your practice progresses. The surface breather, that is to say, is gradually giving way to the authentic breather. You need to do two things: look for what's constant and the same and, at the same time, what's new and different. Try to see your breath through fresh eyes at the start of every practice.

Always be sure to establish yourself in stage 1 before you move along to the higher three stages, even if you're feeling rushed for time. Stage 1 is your foundation. If it's shaky, the house of your breathing practice will topple over in a big, messy pile.

Caution. Recognize that on some days stage 1 will be as far as you get with your practice. If you're not mentally engaged with what you're doing, despite your best intentions, or if your everyday breath seems especially recalcitrant and unwilling to be controlled, then be happy at this stage. While you can strongly encourage yourself to practice on those days when you're feeling reluctant, never force yourself to go beyond stage 1. Not much good will come of it, and tomorrow, as the saying goes, is another day.

Stage 2

Once you're settled down and in contact with your everyday breath, gradually slow your inhales and exhales. On some days you might want to emphasize slow inhale or slow exhale, examining your identity as an inhaler or exhaler much as you do as a breather. In what specific ways does altering just one phase of the breath alter your state of consciousness?

Don't worry at this stage about formal ratio breathing. Allow the slow breathing to find its own cozy ratio. Notice how slowing time affects texture, space, and rest. Often, as you may already have noticed, just by altering one of the qualities, the others are affected as well. Ask yourself again, Who is the breather?

The unspoken mantra will help you to consciously zero in on the qualities of your breath. It also serves as a counterpoint to the silence of the spontaneous rests. Listen carefully to the breathing sounds you make and the intervening silences. Somewhere in there is an important message.

Caution. Just as you did in stage 1, make sure you're established with simple stage 2 slow breathing before you advance to stage 3. This breathing practice, don't forget, is hierarchical. The higher stages are always based on the lower, and the lower must always be in place to support the higher.

Stage 3

Stage 3 is the apex of the daily practice. Along with time, begin to purposely modify texture and space, smoothing and soothing the former and increasing the latter. Initiate ratio breathing, equal ratio first, then unequal ratio, the three bandhas that lock up the openings in the body-pot at the throat and perineum, jalandhara above and modified uddiyana and mula below (see chapter 20).

Caution. More than at stages 1 and 2, exercise caution with your controlled breathing at stage 3. Stay alert for any signs of fatigue, labored breathing, irritability, or headache—anything really that causes upset or discomfort. Never try to push through breathing obstacles, especially early on in your practice. Always stop formal practice and return to everyday breathing at the first indication of trouble.

Stage 4

Last, let go of all control and return to everyday breathing for a few minutes. Notice how, if at all, the formal practice has affected the everyday breathing behavior you contacted in stage 1. Ask yourself again, Who is the breather? After this check-in, lie in Corpse to complete your session.

Conqueror's Breath

Despite the imposing name, Conqueror is a relatively elementary practice. We separate the instruction in this breath, as we do with other breaths in this guide, into its component parts—inhale, exhale, and rest—but that's only for the sake of convenience. In truth, the breathing cycle is an organic whole that can't finally be teased apart without upsetting the delicate breathing balance of taking, giving, and being. As Karlfried Graf Durckheim notes, inhalation is "always the gift of a good exhalation,"[1] and we could add that the reverse is just as true.

PRACTICE: INHALE (PURAKA)

In Sanskrit inhale is *puraka*, which means "filling," "completing," "fulfilling," "satisfying," and also "flood" or "stream." Like life itself, formal pranayama practice always begins on an inhalation.

Which way does your breath move when you breathe? I don't know if this question makes any sense to you, but I've been taught to channel the inhales and exhales vertically through the torso (vertically, that is, in the upright position, parallel to the line of the front spine). Yes, I know, the breath doesn't really move this way: like a lot of instructions in this guide, you can't think too rationally about this one; it's more like one of our "Playing Around" exercises. B. K. S. Iyengar compares this vertical breath, as I call it, to filling a glass with water and emptying it, the water here being the breath and the glass the torso. I've also heard the breath and torso compared to the mercury in a thermometer tube. On the inhale the mercury heats up and rises out of the bulb (in the pelvis), while on the exhale the temperature drops and the mercury falls again.

Draw the inhale, then, upward from the groins along the front spine to the heart, like an elevator rising from the ground floor to the roof of the torso. Spread the sternum and clavicles to receive the breath. Inhale creates a feeling of lightness, as if you were floating up to the ceiling like a balloon.

Each vertical inhale is anchored by lengthening of the tailbone into the floor. As the inhale progresses, maintain this length and the depth of the groins. Make sure, too, that as the inhale reaches its peak in the area of the heart, the hollow at the base of the throat, just above the sternum, stays soft and deep.

There's a little more to learn about Conqueror breathing, which we'll take up in chapter 20.

GOING FURTHER

The breath can be channeled in various directions through and around the torso, not just vertically. Here are two more ways that my students find particularly useful, called cylindrical breath and end-of-twelve breath.

Cylindrical Breath

You can also breathe perpendicularly to the spine (rather than parallel, as in vertical breath). Imagine that your torso is shaped like a cylinder (it's not, but pretend). The axis or altitude of this cylinder is the front spine. If you took a cross section of your torso-cylinder, the axis would be the equivalent of a target's bull's-eye.

Initiate the cylindrical inhale from the entire length of the front spine. Watch it radiate outward from the core of the torso-cylinder to its periphery. I like to imagine cylindrical inhale propagating outward from the front spine like a stack of concentric waves. Then on the exhale the wave returns to its origin in the front spine.

End-of-Twelve Breath

Tradition suggests a third way to channel the breath. I call it the end-of-twelve breath, after an imaginary point outside the body known as the end-of-twelve (dvadasha-anta). This point is twelve fingers' width from the tip of the nose, opposite the heart, where the everyday breath is said to fade away.

First, you have to fix in your imagination the location of the end-of-twelve. Then initiate the inhale from this point and draw the breath into the heart, filling it completely. Next exhale from the heart and imagine the breath streaming back into the outer point again. Yo-yo your breath back and forth between these two points. "If one fixes one's mind at dvadashanta again and again howsoever and wheresoever, the fluctuations of his mind will diminish."[2]

HOW IT HELPS

Inhale is known as the path of action (pravritti-marga). It's the energizing breath, symbolically a reaching out and taking in, an act that animates the body-mind on both the physical and spiritual planes. Inhale is said to flood our being with the universal spirit, a word that in our language shares a common root with several breathing words— inspire and expire, respire and suspire.

The imaginary directions of the vertical, cylindrical, and end-of-twelve exercises help us concentrate our awareness on, and gain another level of control over, the breath.

Caution. Students occasionally ask, How much should I fill the pot on the inhale? All the way or only partway? There are two schools of thought on this issue. One says that you should try to fill the tank fully on the inhale, even to the upper tips of the lungs, which, as I've mentioned, are a bit higher than the level of the clavicles. Many beginning breathers find that topping off the tank in this way creates a lot of tension, which is obviously counterproductive.

The other school recommends, especially for beginners, that you don't inflate the lungs all the way at the end of the inhale. Leaving yourself some breathing room seems to me like a reasonable way to start your pranayama practice. Try inhaling to the level of the eyes of the heart, right below the clavicles. Stop at an even lower level if this feels like too much. Gradually, over weeks and months, increase the amount of air you appropriate on the inhale until you can fill the tank comfortably.

Even when not taking a full inhale, beginners are susceptible to tensing the body. Pay close attention to your breathing barometers, your throat and tongue, eyes, ears, skin of the forehead, and brain. Tension in these places is a dead giveaway that you're overdoing the inhale. Always soften your tongue, eyes, ears, glabella, and brain on the inhale. Focus, too, on the hollow of your throat just above the sternum, what the yogis call the throat well (kantha-kupa). As you inhale, this well should get deeper, not shallower.

Another area where tension is often manifested is in the shoulders. Beginners have a tendency, when sitting for pranayama, to lift their shoulders on the inhale, shortening the neck. Imagine, as you inhale, that your best friend is sitting behind you, resting her hands heavily on your shoulders, weighing them down. Alternatively you could imagine that there are weights hanging from the lower tips of your scapulas. As you inhale, release these weights toward the floor.

If you discover any of these warning signs of an inhale struggle, and you can't release them despite your best efforts, stop your practice immediately and return to everyday breathing. Then back off slightly the next time you breathe. Don't rush the lions, elephants, and tigers.

PRACTICE: EXHALE (RECHAKA)

Exhale is *rechaka*, "emptying." Formal pranayama practice always ends, just as does life, with an exhale. We've mostly covered vertical, cylindrical, and end-of-twelve exhale in the inhale practice. But there are a few more things we can say about exhalation.

I've already said quite a bit about exhale in the inhale practice. Vertical exhale is like pouring the water out of our imaginary glass or cooling off the mercury in the thermometer or punching the ground-floor button in the elevator.

Begin the exhale from the lifted heart. On the exhale beginning breathers tend to sink the front of their torso, much as a blow-up toy will sag when its air is let out. Just before you begin the exhale, open the eyes of the heart wide in wonder and amazement. Remember to support the lift of the heart by firming the scapulas against the back ribs and lengthening the front spine.

Just as the inhale is anchored by the descent of the tailbone into the center of the earth, so is the exhale anchored by the eyes of the heart. Maintain this openness for as long as you can without hardening the chest. I sometimes imagine there's a tiny yogi helper inside my heart, pushing with all her might on the inside of my sternum, holding it high as my breath departs. Eventually these eyes will close, but make that happen slowly and softly.

B. K. S. Iyengar mentions somewhere—and I've lost this source in the haze of bad memory—that we should exhale "reluctantly." I've always appreciated this word. It seems as if he's asking us to consciously savor each breath to the fullest, as if it were our last, which is, I believe, the essence of the pranayama.

In the sitting position, finish the exhale by burrowing the tailbone down into the floor and deepening the groins. Imagine that your tail, normally curled slightly inward toward the pubis, is uncurling like one of those party favors that, when you blow into the mouthpiece, whistles and unrolls a spool of paper—except that your coccyx won't whistle. The long tail then anchors the next inhale. Pretend that, as the breath is rising along the front spine to the heart, it's counterbalanced by the tail diving into the heart of the planet, almost four thousand miles away. In this fashion vertical breath follows and supports the spinal circuit of up-the-front and down-the-back.

HOW IT HELPS

Exhale is the path of cessation (nivritti-marga), the calming breath. It represents letting go, a willing surrender of the surface self, what Karlfried Graf Durckheim describes as a "leap into the unknown with total confidence and without restrictions, developing the receptivity of the seeker in the extreme."[3]

When you consciously extend the time of your exhale, you automatically encourage the time of the inhale to extend as well. A reluctant exhale increases the uptake of oxygen, so that breathing becomes more efficient, and helps calm the brain, which is especially conducive to relieving stress and stilling those restless fluctuations of citta.

Caution. Make sure that you don't simply jut the front ribs forward to help lift the heart eyes. This merely tenses the chest and shortens the lower back, restricting the movement of the roots of the diaphragm.

PRACTICE: REST (VISHRAMA)

Rest is vishrama, "repose," "relaxation," "calm," "tranquility," and also a "resting place," a "pause." You could say that rest is the goal of classical yoga. When we rest or restrict, as Patanjali puts it, our body in asana, our breath in retention, our senses in sense-withdrawal, and the fluctuations of our surface self in meditation and samadhi, then and only then do we abide, as Patanjali concludes, in our essence or own true form (sva-rupa). When the knower, writes the Kashmiri sage Somananda, "no longer discovers any other object to be known [apart from himself] and when his energy rests in Shiva, that is called 'repose.'"[4]

The two breathing rests, inner and outer, are natural retentions, and the two retentions (kumbhaka) are nothing more than a prolongation—at first willful, then spontaneous—of the everyday rests. Early on in your Conqueror practice, simply witness the two everyday rests. Do nothing to purposely extend them. Remember that by just by slowing the time of the breath, the rests, too, will slow. (We'll work with the willful retention of the breath in chapter 20.)

HOW IT HELPS

Notice what happens to your citta during these brief rests. The movement of the everyday inhales and exhales feeds the vrittis. But during the rests, the vrittis are momentarily cut off from their food supply, so to speak. If they don't exactly come to a full stop—they are still, after all, nourished by our unconscious—they at least slow down. We can, if we're quick enough, catch a break between one thought and the next and a glimpse, however fleeting, of what Patanjali means by citta-vritti-nirodha, the restriction of the fluctuations of consciousness. Then the challenge is to fix ourselves in that moment of stillness.

PLAYING AROUND: CONQUEROR BREAK

While Conqueror is traditionally a formal practice performed in the sitting position, you can take short Conqueror breaks throughout your day. Wherever you are, whenever you have a quiet moment or two, sit comfortably, close your eyes, and perform a mini-Conqueror. When you have some experience with the breath, you might even try it while you're walking. One of my students reports that, when she's out for a walk in the hills behind her house, the breath helps her conquer the uphill climbs.

LAST WORD

We're often warned of the rigors and demands of yoga and its associated practices, and in this guide we've responded by taking a purposely cautious approach to pranayama. But it seems to me that in the end nothing very difficult is asked of us. We have all the tools for our own self-realization right at hand—in the body, the breath, and the sound of our voice—and the entire process may not be as daunting as it sounds.

CHAPTER 19

Against-the-Grain Breath
Viloma Pranayama

The function of stopping is to achieve a more differentiated and refined action. It is also meant to prolong a gesture, to perpetuate a connection or relationship so that
more learning can occur.

—Stanley Kelemann, *Embodying Experience*

The possibility of a pause between the creation of a
thought pattern for any particular action and the execution
of that action is the physical basis for awareness. This pause
makes it possible to examine what is happening within us
at the moment when the intention to act is formed as well
as when it is carried out. The possibility of delaying action—
prolonging the period between the intention and its execution—enables man to know himself.

—Moishe Feldenkrais, *Awareness Through Movement*

VILOMA PRANAYAMA isn't mentioned in the traditional guides, and
in many modern guides the name is given to a practice very different from the one described here. This version of viloma is based on the
teaching of B. K. S. Iyengar.

Viloma means "against (vi) the hair or grain (loma)," "contrary
to the usual or proper course." This means viloma is contrary to the
usual course of everyday breathing, in which the inhales and exhales
are more or less continuous from beginning to end. Against-the-
Grain is a stop-and-go or interrupted breath, in which the inhales
and exhales are done in brief steps, separated by equally brief rests.

Against-the-Grain continues and completes your work with zigzag breathing (chapter 12). As I mentioned, the reverse breaths of zigzag are replaced here with brief rests.

Four Stages of Daily Practice

If you've done your homework with unusual breathing (chapter 12), particularly zigzag breathing, then Against-the-Grain will be a breeze. Like Conqueror with the first three unusual-breathing exercises, Against-the-Grain is the fulfillment or completion of zigzag breathing.

PRELIMINARY

Reread the "Preliminary" section for Conqueror (chapter 18). For viloma you'll need to decide which one of the three marking techniques discussed later in the chapter—Time Against-the-Grain, Space Against-the-Grain, or Time-and-Space Against-the-Grain—you'll be using for the practice.

Stage 1

The instructions and caution for stage 1 Against-the-Grain are the same as those for Conqueror.

Stage 2

Once you're settled down and in contact with your everyday breath, begin to gradually break or interrupt your inhales and exhales. Just to keep the lions, elephants, and tigers happy, I recommend that, for the first few weeks of your practice with this breath, you do the inhales and exhales separately. Do inhales on even-numbered days, exhales on odd, or if you have the time, inhales first in your daily practice session, then exhales. When this is comfortable, join the inhales and exhales along with the rests into a complete four-phase viloma cycle. Then over time increase the number of breaks in the breath.

Listen carefully to the unspoken mantra. I particularly enjoy the music in the alteration of SA or HA and the intervening silences. Try to anchor yourself in the stillness between and underneath the breaths. What happens to the fluctuations in the silences? See if you can maintain that state even during the inhales and exhales.

Stage 3

Now apply any techniques your schedule calls for, such as Lower Belly Lock or prolonged inner retention at the end of the last step of your inhale (see chapter 20). Work, too, with Against-the-Grain in conjunction with Conqueror. There are various ways you can combine the two breaths. Early on in your breathing career, do Conqueror first, then Against-the-Grain. But when you get some experience with these two breaths, you can periodically reverse the order of the two; or do Conqueror, then Against-the-Grain, then Conqueror again; or spend an entire session on Against-the-Grain.

Stage 4

Last, return to everyday breathing. Let go of all control and notice how, if at all, the pranayama has affected your everyday breathing behavior. Ask yourself again, Who is the breather? After this check-in, lie in Corpse to complete your session.

Against-the-Grain Breath

Against-the-Grain is certainly a more complicated affair than Conqueror. That's why it's best to gain some facility with the latter before you take a crack at the former. It's not uncommon for students to get hung up with Against-the-Grain. If you suddenly feel confused or clumsy, unable to smoothly coordinate the transition of the breath from one step to the next, don't worry—you're not alone.

Over the years I've been taught two ways to breathe against the grain. I call them Time Against-the-Grain and Space Against-the-Grain.

PRACTICE: TIME AGAINST-THE-GRAIN

Each inhale, rest, and exhale matches a short count, most often two or three. Usually the counts are equal ratio—for example, two-to-two or three-to-three. As a beginning breather, though, it's acceptable to make the inhale or exhale slightly longer than the rest—say, two-to-one.

Caution. You might not be able to breathe with Time Against-the-Grain continuously throughout your entire practice.

PRACTICE: SPACE AGAINST-THE-GRAIN

Each step of the inhale fills, and each step of the exhale empties, successive sections of the torso or thorax and lungs, so that your breath moves up or down as if climbing or descending a ladder rung by rung similarly to vertical breathing. While Time Against-the-Grain breaks the breath into relatively equal steps based on counts, Space Against-the-Grain is based more on feel, and so the inhales, exhales, and rests may not be exactly equal.

There are various ways to divide the torso or rib case for Space Against-the-Grain, depending on how much detail you want to work with. Keep it fairly simple at first. For example, you can divide the rib case horizontally at the midsternum. On the first inhale-step, fill the area from the bottom of the rib case to this line, and on the second fill the area above the line to the collarbones. Once you're accustomed to this two-step practice, you can parse the rib case into three or even four sections. For example:

- From the floating ribs to the false ribs
- From the false ribs to the bottom of the sternum
- From the bottom of the sternum to the armpits
- From the armpits to the clavicles

You can also divide and breathe into the entire torso. For example, you might chop up the torso from the pubis to the navel, from the navel to the bottom of the sternum, from the bottom of the sternum to the line of the nipples, and from the line of the nipples to the top of the shoulders.

GOING FURTHER

Once you've mastered some of the simpler divisions of the rib case or torso, feel free to experiment with other, more complicated Against-the-Grain spaces. You could, for example, quarter the entire torso again, then breathe only into the right-side spaces for five to ten cycles, then repeat the exercise with the left-side spaces for an equal number of cycles. There's nothing to stop you from making up some spaces of your own, even including spaces in the hands and feet or, if you're feeling really adventurous, somewhere outside the body.

Experiment, too, with the direction of the movement of the inhales and exhales. You can work both vertically, from bottom to top or top to bottom, and cylindrically, from the core to the periphery or from the periphery to the core.

HOW IT HELPS

Against-the-Grain helps to intensify breath awareness and improve breath control (ayama). Breathing is a process, and each breath—whether inhale or exhale—has a beginning, a middle, and an end and is always followed by a moment of rest and reflection. By resting and reflecting at selected points along the way—according to time, space, or time-and-space—we can take a closer look at the various stages in the process of breathing, to learn more about their particulars and peculiarities. The rests are little retentions that have (as you'll learn in chapter 20) a calming effect on our fluctuations. Against-the-Grain is, then, also a preparation for full retention.

Caution. As I mentioned before, some aspirants report that Space Against-the-Grain is frustrating because they can't quite coordinate the movement of the breath through the variously defined layers of the torso. Be sure not to start your practice of Space Against-the-Grain too ambitiously and divide yourself up into too many layers.

Two layers, as I described above, should give you more than enough to work with for the first few weeks of your practice.

PLAYING AROUND: SPONTANEOUS AGAINST-THE-GRAIN

The breathing steps and rests in Time Against-the-Grain and Space Against-the-Grain are more or less formal or determined, either by a set count or by a predefined area of the body. With spontaneous Against-the-Grain, though, your breathing steps sort of "go with the flow," to use a popular phrase.

For this exercise I'll describe only inhale Against-the-Grain, though the same instructions apply to the exhale. Start the cycle, as always, with a full exhalation. Then begin the first step of your vertical inhale at the base of the pelvis. Don't count or direct the breath into any particular area. Keep on just until you begin to feel the effort or tension of the body, whether that's in the groins, heart, throat, brain, wherever. Then stop and rest for as long as you need in order to release as much of the effort or tension, wherever you locate it, as you can. One student reported that he needed long rests early on in the session, up to about ten counts, but that the rests grew briefer as the session progressed.

Once you feel this release, begin the second step of the inhale. Again, go along until the effort or tension returns, whether in the same place (or places) or in a new place (or places), and rest again. Proceed in this fashion, inhaling neither to a count nor to an area. The only determinant of the time and space of the inhale-step is your own response to it. Each step may be long or short, and none of the steps may match. Stop stepping upward when you feel comfortably full of breath, then slowly exhale.

HOW IT HELPS

Even at this late date in the practice, some students still chafe when asked to impose an artificial pattern on the breath. Playing around by acknowledging your own reactions to the breath and integrating them into the practice serves as an excellent counterpoint to the demands of formal practice.

LAST WORD

Against-the-Grain is a powerful reminder that breathing is an inter-play between action and nonaction. It gives us the opportunity to witness the movement of our breath against the universal backdrop of absolute stillness.

CHAPTER 20

Locks and Retention
Bandha and Kumbhaka

When the Shakti in the form of exhalation is retained outside (at dvadashanta), and in the form of inhalation is retained inside (at the hrt or heart center), then at the end of this practice [of retention, or kumbhaka], the Shakti is known as Shanta or tranquillized and through Shakti Shanta the divine self (Bhairava) is revealed.

—Vijnana-Bhairava, "Meditation 4," in *The Yoga of Delight, Wonder, and Astonishment*, translated by Jaideva Singh

Locks (Bandha)

It isn't widely recognized that Hatha-Yoga includes, in addition to asana and pranayama, a third essential category of practices, composed of locks (bandha) and seals (mudra). They're said to cure various diseases and "destroy" death, increase the gastric fire, restrain and channel vital energy in the torso and intensify its transformative potency, confer miraculous powers, and awaken kundalini and lead to samadhi and liberation.

It's difficult to succinctly characterize these widely varied practices, but in general they're muscular contractions or asanalike positions; pressurings of two body parts (for example, the chin to the chest, the heel to the perineum, the tongue to the palate); and even meditations (dharana) on traditional elements, like earth or fire, localized in the body.

Three of the most important bandhas for pranayama are called Root Lock (mula-bandha), Net-Bearer Lock (jalandhara-bandha), and Upward Lock (uddiyana-bandha). Root Lock is a contraction of the muscles at the root of the pelvis that locks the anus and perineum, while Net-Bearer Lock is a pressuring of the chin and sternum that locks the throat. Together they have two functions: they close the two openings of the alimentary canal so the vital breath can't leak out of the pot, and they join and concentrate the forces of apana-vayu and prana-vayu (see chapter 2), which normally flow in opposite directions (there's another esoteric purpose for Net-Bearer, which I'll go into later). "Raising the apana upward and bringing the prana down from the throat, the yogi becomes free from old age and appears as if sixteen years of age."[1]

In Upward Lock the abdominal muscles are contracted and sucked up and into the abdominal cavity toward the spine. This churns and heats the consolidated vayus, which the yogis then use to rouse kundalini and swing wide the gate to liberation.

In this chapter we'll work with Net-Bearer Lock; a lock that's akin to Upward Lock, which I call Lower Belly Lock; and a modified Root Lock. Upward and Root Lock proper are considered to be more advanced practices best learned under the supervision of an experienced teacher.

Net-Bearer Lock (*Jalandhara-bandha*)

Jalandhara-bandha is performed by pressing the lowered chin to the raised sternum. It's the natural companion of the Lower Belly and Root Locks, sealing off the head end of the torso-pot.

While the Sanskrit name is commonly interpreted as "chin lock" or "throat lock," neither is a literal translation. Jalandhara is composed of two words, jala (spelled and pronounced with a long first a) and dhara. Jala is a "net for catching birds," "web," "mesh," or "snare," and dhara means "bearing," "supporting," as well as a "vein" or "tubular vessel of the body." Literally jalandhara-bandha is the "Net-Bearer Lock."

By this the yogis imply that the lock bears down on or squeezes the net of channels, both coarse and subtle, in the neck in order to regulate the currents of blood and prana circulating to the heart, the thyroid gland, and the organs of the head (especially the eyes, ears, and brain) and to guard them from sudden surges of energy.

Be aware that the names chin lock and throat lock can be misleading. Chin lock seems to imply that jalandhara is fixed solely by the chin's pressing on the sternum. But this is only half the equation. The chin does drop toward the sternum, but in order to avoid overstretching and injuring the muscles of the back of the neck, the sternum must equally lift up toward the chin. Maybe a more accurate way to describe the bandha would be the chin-sternum lock.

Also, the English word lock could be misconstrued, because it unfortunately conjures up the notion that Net-Bearer is clamped down like a padlock. Most of us already hold too much tension in our throat, which interferes with the easy flow of everyday breathing. Increasing that tension with a rigid Net-Bearer could have unhappy consequences, like headaches, dizziness, and irritability. I'll talk more about how and how not to work with jalandhara properly in the practice sections that follow.

Net-Bearer Lock is for sitters only.

PRELIMINARY

To work on this lock, you'll need one or two folded blankets, a rolled elastic bandage or washcloth, a metal folding chair, and any other props you like for Chair Seat.

Before attempting Net-Bearer Lock, reacquaint yourself with the root of the neck (in chapter 14) and the hyoid-atlas-inion circuit (in chapter 9). Lie down again in Bridge posture, with the sharp edge of the blanket(s) pressing against the root of your neck. Your head and neck will be in flexion, with the chin near, or even against, the manubrium.

As you did in the Bridge exercise, lift from the neck root diagonally through the torso to the manubrium, without pushing the lower front ribs toward the ceiling. Press your fingertips lightly against the horns of the hyoid and, as the crook of the neck deepens, watch the bone lift diagonally through the skull, across the atlas to the inion. Release the inion away from the nape and the nape toward the scapulas.

Now connect the two circuits. From the neck root lift to the manubrium, from the manubrium to the hyoid, from the hyoid across the atlas to the inion. At the inion release down the back to the neck root, where the circuit begins again. Witness this energy circuit for a few minutes.

PRACTICE

Sit in the Chair Seat with whatever props you like. Start with your head upright. As the back spine descends to the coccyx, lift diagonally from the neck root to the sternum and initiate the manubrium-hyoid-atlas-inion circuit. Then, and only then, pivot the chin and elongate it downward over the hyoid and drop it toward the sternum (see fig. 20.1).

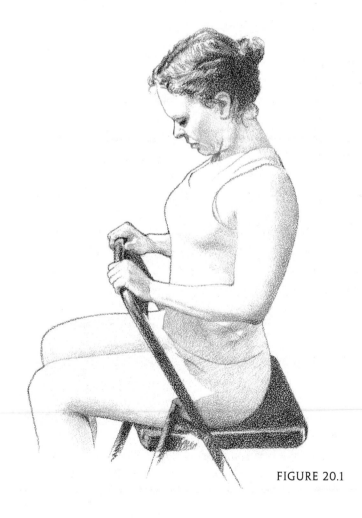

FIGURE 20.1

HOW IT HELPS

Theos Bernard writes that Net-Bearer is a "simple technique used to prevent the air from rushing up into the head" and, along with its companion locks, helps confine "the air within the body and create an abdominal pressure. The purpose assigned to this pressure is that it enables one to control the breath at will and thus to gain control of the mind."[2] According to Alain Danielou, the Net-Bearer pressures the purity wheel (vishuddha-chakra) in the throat, which is a kind of command station for the network of perception-transmitting nerves in the body. The contraction "protects the ends of the nerves from the brutal pressure of the air while holding the breath."[3]

Bernard also maintains that Net-Bearer creates an upward pull on the spinal cord, which, in turn, affects the brain. In this sense jala refers to the brain and the nerve, which he doesn't specify, passing through the neck, and dhara denotes the upward pull.

This nerve might be related to what Swami Rama calls the channel of consciousness, or vijnani-nadi. The Net-Bearer compresses the carotid arteries, which feed blood to the brain; this, in turn, slows the heartbeat and protects the heart from the stresses of kumbhaka.

I mentioned earlier that there's an esoteric purpose for Net-Bearer. The yogis report that some of the nadis are pipelines for an elixir of immortality called juice (soma) or immortal (amrita), exuded by a center located sometimes in the brain, other times in the throat. In the average human, this liquid drips into the belly and is burned up in the fires of the solar plexus. Because of this, Svatmarama notes, the body ages and eventually dies. Net-Bearer dams up the pipelines that pass through the neck and preserves the elixir. It's in this sense that Bernard calls it the "receptacle of vital fluid."[4]

I've found that Net-Bearer encourages me to lift the top of my sternum—using the lowered chin as a tactile aid—as well as the front of the spine, the energetic core of my torso. This action does two things: it helps me to open the eyes of the chest and the upper lobes of the lungs, enlarging my breathing capacity; and it sharpens my awareness of my body's central axis, which then serves to organize and anchor my sitting position.

Also, with my head bowed in a gesture of contemplation and my eyes directed downward toward this core, Net-Bearer helps to draw my otherwise scattered awareness inward and calm the incessant fluctuations of citta.

Caution. Net-Bearer should be used with caution, especially if you have neck problems. Never force your chin to the sternum. Be sure also to bring the chin straight down to the middle of the manubrium and don't angle it off to one side. Keep what the yogis call the throat well (kantha-kupa), the little hollow at the top of the sternum, soft and deep throughout this practice.

GOING FURTHER

For the first few weeks or months of your practice of Net-Bearer, don't hold the lock continuously throughout your practice session but only for the retention and the exhale. Also, don't create the lock and retain the breath after every inhale. Intersperse two to three rounds of ujjayi without retention between each kumbhaka.

It's likely that your chin won't reach, or at least won't comfortably reach, the sternum. To avoid straining your neck muscles, B. K. S. Iyengar instructs beginning Net-Bearers to support the chin on, and lift the sternum against, a firmly rolled-up bandage or washcloth (see fig. 20.2).

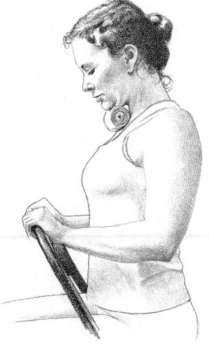

FIGURE 20.2

The bandage does present one small problem. Each time you raise your head at the end of the exhale, the roll will fall in your lap unless you hold it in place with your hand. I find this distracting. So I secure the roll by sliding it under the edge of my T-shirt collar or, in winter, by snugging it in the folds of my favorite turtleneck practice shirt.

As your practice develops, you can gradually make the roll smaller and smaller, until you can do the lock without it. But as with all of the practices in this guide, don't be in a hurry.

Be sure to work on the neck root–manubrium-hyoid-atlas-inion circuit in your asana practice. The best asana to improve your Net-Bearer practice is Shoulderstand (sarvangasana) and all its variations.

Modified Lower Belly Lock (Uddiyana-bandha)

Lower Belly Lock is my name for a moderate firmness of the lower belly muscle during inhalation. This firmness is created not so much by forcefully contracting and gripping the muscle itself as by subtly working around the area of the lower belly to:

- Center the femur heads in the hip sockets and deepen the groins
- Narrow the front of the pelvis and widen the back
- Narrow and lift the skin of the lower belly toward the navel while lengthening the tail downward
- Shift the weight or mass of the lower belly diagonally up and into the abdominal cavity

Most of these actions are familiar to you from your mapping expedition and your practice of the asanas.

PRACTICE: RECLINING LOWER BELLY LOCK

We'll learn this lock in a reclining position and then, after an appropriate length of time, move to a sitting position.

You'll need a round bolster or rolled blanket and whatever props you like for Bent-Knee Corpse. You could also use two sandbags.

Lie in Bent-Knee Corpse. If you have two sandbags, lay them across the creases of your groins, so that they form a V with its apex at your pubis. As you know, during everyday breathing, the belly muscle (rectus abdominis) relaxes and puffs on the inhale, as the diaphragm contracts and descends against the organs, and contracts on the exhale, as the diaphragm relaxes and pushes up into the thorax. Witness this up-and-down movement of the lower belly for a few minutes. Use your fingertips for tactile aids if needed.

Drop your femur heads away from the weight of the bags toward the back of your pelvis and draw the inner groins up into the torso and feed them into the front spine. Use your fingertips to press your two hip points closer together, so the front of the pelvis narrows and the back widens. Hold for a minute or so. Then slide your fingertips onto the lower belly and push the sides of the muscle inward, toward its midline and the navel, and upward, from the pubis toward the navel. Lengthen your tail along the floor toward your heels.

Now imagine there's a weight, like a water-filled balloon, inside your lower belly. Sink this weight away from the rectus muscle and down onto the sacrum, as you continue to widen the bone to accept the weight. No matter how long you stay with this exercise, the weight will never actually touch the back of your pelvis but will go on sinking, at least to the end of your current incarnation. Then lift the weight lightly away from your perineum toward your diaphragm.

For the next few minutes, with everyday breathing, watch how these actions tend to slightly firm and hollow the lower belly and the perineum into the abdominal cavity, even during your inhales, when normally the belly would puff. Don't apply this lock to your actual pranayama practice until you can do it consistently and confidently with everyday breathing.

Feel free to use your hands as tactile aids. Touch your fingertips lightly to the lower belly and use them to monitor the quality of the lock.

Caution. Though I've already mentioned it, I'll remind you again not to perform this lock by hardening your lower belly muscle. In this guide Lower Belly Lock is created indirectly through what are, in the end, mostly imaginative actions. In the early stages of your practice, use this lock cautiously. Release as much tension from your lower belly as you can before you practice. The Belly Roll and Bridge exercises (chapter 14) can help you do this.

Always practice Lower Belly Lock on an empty stomach

GOING FURTHER

When you're ready to apply the lock to your formal practice, begin Conqueror breathing proper. Exhale and, on the ensuing inhale, lock the lower belly against the descending diaphragm, which is pressuring the abdominal organs to push outward. Remember that you're locking only the lower belly on the inhale, not the upper belly (above the navel and below the xiphoid), which should continue to puff. You can touch your fingertips on this area for tactile aid to make sure there's no hardness. Notice how, if at all, this resistance in the lower belly changes the qualities of the inhale. Continue the lock for a few minutes more, taking an unlocked inhale whenever needed.

PRACTICE: SITTING LOWER BELLY LOCK

Sitting Lower Belly Lock is created with the same actions as its reclining version. When you were supine, though, with the pull of gravity at your back, it was relatively easy to sink and lift the weight of your belly. Now, sitting upright, you're working against gravity, so this imaginative action might take you a little more time and effort to establish.

For the sitting version of Lower Belly Lock, you'll require a folding chair and whatever props you like for Chair Seat, along with a rolled-up sticky mat or towel and a strap, buckled into a large loop.

Sit in Chair Seat with your loop and sticky mat within reach. Slide through the chair until your lower belly is touching the front of the chair back. Slip the loop over your feet and legs and up onto your midthighs. Parallel your thighs and snug the loop around them. The strap will prevent your legs from falling apart and keep your groins soft. Be sure not to let the thighs press outward heavily against the strap.

Wedge the rolled-up mat between the chair legs and your lower belly. Rest your hands on your thighs or on the chair back. As you did in your reclining practice, witness the movement of the lower belly for a few minutes in everyday breathing, with the sticky mat as a tactile aid. Feel how the belly bulges into and then firms away from the mat as you inhale and exhale.

Now re-create the actions in the pelvis, groins, and lower belly described for the reclining version. Drop your femur heads into the pelvis and sharpen the inner groins, use your hands to narrow the hip points and widen the sacrum, and lift the skin of the lower belly from the pubis to the navel. Uncurl your tail through an imaginary hole in the chair seat and down onto the floor.

Now draw your belly weight away from the rolled mat toward your sacrum, then lift it away from the pelvic floor. Again, notice how this lift, as well as contributing to the Belly Lock, also sucks the perineum up lightly into the pelvis.

For the next few minutes, with everyday breathing, watch how these actions tend to slightly firm and hollow the lower belly and the perineum into the abdominal cavity, even during your inhales, when normally the belly would puff. Don't apply this lock to your actual pranayama practice until you can do it consistently and confidently with everyday breathing.

HOW IT HELPS

Remember that in everyday inhalation the descending diaphragm pushes against the viscera, which, in turn, push against the belly muscle, which relaxes and balloons. Applied during pranayama inhalation, the lock sets up a breathing chain reaction: the firmed lower belly resists the pressure of the viscera, and the viscera, in turn, resist the downward movement of the diaphragm. Since it's now prevented from descending fully into the belly, the diaphragm instead expands the rib case much more than usual. This encourages the breath to move higher, into the upper chest around the eyes of the heart, enlivening the upper tips of the lungs, which are often dull.

Over time the lock also helps massage the viscera and tone the lower belly muscle. The muscle then becomes a more efficient pump for the exhale, which helps to clean out the lungs and aid the return of blood to the heart, thereby lightening its workload.

Caution. The cautions for the reclining lock apply to the sitting version as well.

GOING FURTHER

When you're ready to apply the lock to your formal practice, begin Conqueror breathing proper. Run through the same instructions as you did with the reclining version.

Modified Root Lock (Mula-bandha)

Once you're comfortable with Lower Belly Lock, you can work with a variation of Root Lock (mula-bandha). Root Lock lifts the base of the pelvis, as if sucking the perineum up into the torso. In this guide, though, this action isn't created forcefully by contracting the perineal muscles. Here we'll induce the lock using only our imagination and, if you're game, a simple prop.

PRACTICE

You'll need as props a tennis ball or some other similarly shaped, relatively soft object, like a rolled-up elastic bandage. Imagine that your breath is attached to the base of your pelvis with a long string. As the breath is drawn upward along the front spine on the inhale, watch this string slowly tautening and tugging the perineum gently along, doming it into the pelvis. During the inhale, pause and feel the firmness at the base of your pelvis and lower belly. Maintain this firmness as much as you can for as long as you can on the exhale, then release it and loosen the perineum and belly during the exhale rest.

You can't use your hands here, as you did on your belly, as tactile aids. So to give myself a touch at the perineum, I like to sit—lightly, as you might guess—with a tennis ball against my perineum. The ball helps create the dome shape on the perineum.

HOW IT HELPS

As I've mentioned, traditionally Root Lock, along with its companion locks, works to seal the torso-pot, to prevent any prana from leaking out through the throat or anus. It also helps to raise the normally downward-flowing apana-vayu (see chapter 2) toward the base of the spine, where it can be concentrated to assist in the awakening of kundalini.

Caution. Again, as with Lower Belly Lock, don't perform Root Lock by tightening the muscles at the base of your pelvis. This may be the traditional way to execute the lock, but it's not recommended at this still-early stage of your pranayama practice, especially without the supervision of a teacher. Release as much tension from your perineum as you can before you practice. The two variations of Reclining Bound Angle posture (chapter 14) are very effective preparations.

Retention (Kumbhaka)

The practice of retention, or kumbhaka, seems strange to many of my beginning breathers. Whenever I talk about breath holding, I can always count on at least a few incredulous stares. They ask me, "But isn't it unnatural, even dangerous, to hold your breath?" They wonder, too, why it is that the journey of the yoga of breathing ends with . . . not breathing.

Actually it's not so strange for us to stop breathing. We spontaneously do it all the time, when we feel surprised or in danger. Breathing stops so it doesn't distract us from looking closely at what's surprising or dangerous, and so we don't make unnecessary sounds or movements to attract unwanted attention.

You could say that the yogis stop breathing for a somewhat similar reason. Everyday breathing, according to Patanjali, helps sustain the fluctuations of the surface self and its avidya, which distracts the aspirant from concentrated looking for his authentic self. When breathing stops in kumbhaka, so do some, though not all, of the fluctuations, and the veil that obscures the looking is partially lifted.

I guess it might be better not to say that you stop breathing in kumbhaka. The average person, without training in pranayama, obviously shouldn't—and probably couldn't—stop breathing for more than a couple of minutes. Kumbhaka, though, is a special kind of stopping, only performed when the aspirant has rigorously trained himself to tap into the very essence of life, the infinite pranic reservoir of the universe. For the average person, breathing is an end in itself—without it he can't survive. But for the yogi what we understand as breathing is a means to an end, a tool that both increases and conserves the aspirant's vital energy, and intensifies and channels its transformative power. In kumbhaka, while the outer movements of breathing stop (they're a distraction and a waste of energy), the inner subtle breathing continues. Far from being strange, you could say that kumbhaka is really the completion or perfection of all breathing.

PRELIMINARY

There are two traditional forms of kumbhaka: inner retention (antar-kumbhaka), which follows the inhale, and outer retention (bahya-kumbhaka), which follows the exhale. We'll work only with inner retention in this guide. Like the formal Root and Upward Locks, outer retention is a relatively advanced practice best learned under the guidance of an experienced teacher. For the time being, to work with outer retention, simply prolong the everyday outer rest for three to four counts.

PRACTICE: INNER RETENTION (ANTAR-KUMBHAKA)

Retention is appropriate only for sitters in either the Chair Seat or traditional seats, not recliners. Recliners should attend to and prolong for three or four counts the inner and outer rests as a preparation for formal sitting retention. Don't try long retentions until you're competent in viloma pranayama and the Net-Bearer and Lower Belly Locks.

We'll learn inner retention with ujjayi breathing in Chair Seat, then transfer what you learn to traditional sitting. So you'll need a metal folding chair and whatever other props you like for Chair Seat. If needed, also have a rolled elastic bandage as a support for Net-Bearer Lock.

Sit in Chair Seat and establish your best equal ratio count. For this example we'll say that's six counts. Then start off—as all lions, elephants, and tigers do—conservatively with a three count for retention.

As you near the end of the six-count inhale, initiate Net-Bearer Lock from the root of the neck (and apply the modified Lower Belly and Root Locks), so that as breath comes to its end, the chin and sternum, with or without the intervening rolled bandage, meet. Retain the breath for three counts. Hold the torso steady with a long front spine. Lift the diaphragm to support the lungs and heart.

Gradually increase the time of your retention in sama-vritti. This may take a few days, weeks, months, or years. Aim to match the retention count to the inhale-exhale count, so that the ratio is one-to-one-to-one. Traditionally the recommended count for the retention is ultimately four times that of the inhale—that is, one-to-four. Approach this ratio with all due caution.

Once you've reached the one-to-one-to-one ratio in sama-vritti, you can begin to work with vishama-vritti. Start out again with an inner retention of half the inhale count and again gradually increase it until it matches the inhale count. Proceed beyond this point with caution.

As you retain the breath, circulate the locked-in prana throughout the entire torso.

Maintain the Net-Bearer Lock during the exhale. Then, when the exhale is done, lift your head back to upright. Take three or four rounds of ujjayi without retention. Repeat this sequence for the length of your practice session.

HOW IT HELPS

For our purposes retention is a willfully prolonged rest in the breathing cycle that allows us to extract the maximum amount of prana from the inhaled air and soak it into all the cells of our body. This both calms and invigorates the body-mind, stretches and strengthens our breathing muscles and lungs, and makes us more efficient breathers. It helps us direct awareness away from the outside world and toward the inner world of our authentic self. Inhales and exhales are fluctuations that bind us to the everyday world of becoming. When we stop these fluctuations in kumbhaka, the grip of this world, and its avidya, is loosened. We become more like our authentic self, still and serene, self-contained, joyful.

Caution. Make sure you don't grip the breath with your body during retention. This tends to harden just about everything. You want especially to keep the tongue, eyes, ears, and brain soft during retention. As you're learning to hold your breath, you might want to wrap your forehead with an elastic bandage (see chapter 10) and shrink your brain to the back of your skull.

One aspirant wrote in her journal that breath holding caused her to panic. "I feel like I won't be able to breathe again or get enough air again." Be sure not to let your retention get to this point. Build up your time slowly in the tradition of the lions, elephants, and tigers. It helps, when you're first learning retention, to take three to four ujjayi breaths without retentions between every breath with retention. Then over time, as you increase the length of your retentions, gradually decrease the number of the intervening nonretention cycles.

Students with high blood pressure should avoid retention, unless supervised by an experienced teacher.

LAST WORD

Here we are at the last Last Word, and thank goodness for that because I'm pretty much out of useful information. Let me just add a few practice reminders to send you on your way. Periodically reevaluate your breathing practice in the context of your larger spiritual efforts. Ask yourself, Why am I doing this? Recognize and value the short-term physical benefits of the practice, but always keep in the back of your mind the ultimate goal of the work, what Patanjali calls the vision of the self (purusha-khyati).

Always keep your practice within comfortable limits. Remember that the breath—like lions, elephants, and tigers—should be tamed slowly. Stay with a particular breath, or an aspect of the breath, for a good long while. Get to know your breath intimately so that you live with it moment to moment. Be willing, though, at times, to experiment, to go out on a limb and take a risk.

Remember, too, that change in the breath comes slowly. As Westerners, we're committed to the idea of a linear kind of progress, as if our practice should move inexorably in a straight line from point A to point B. That probably won't happen as you travel through the country of the Self—at least that hasn't been my experience over the last eighteen or so years. Things go smoothly for a while, then come to a dead stop, start up all over again, then go straight downhill, all with no apparent logical explanation.

It might happen that, despite your best efforts, you simply can't bring yourself to practice pranayama. It doesn't mean you're a bad person. Just let it go and put this guide on the shelf in a safe place. Stay with your asana practice, taking care to end each session with a ten- to fifteen-minute Corpse. This will help you to lay the foundation for the practice when the time is ripe for you to resume. As Krishna reminds Arjuna in the Gita:

> No effort in this world
> is lost or wasted;
> a fragment of sacred duty
> saves you from great fear.[5]

Shivam.
May there be good to all!

APPENDIX 1

Practice Schedule Outline

MOST YOGA instructional guides include some kind of practice schedule for their users. These schedules are generally of two kinds. The first we could call a fixed schedule, in which the practice sequences and the time frame of the practice are spelled out in definite terms. All you have to do every day is look at the schedule, and it will tell you exactly what to do and for how long. The second kind of schedule is more flexible and open-ended. Here the teacher provides only a bare outline for the work and leaves it up to the student to fill in the day-to-day details.

There are advantages and disadvantages to each of these kinds of schedules. One big problem with the fixed schedule, of course, is that not everybody progresses at the same rate. Some people can follow along just fine according to the recommended sequences and time frame, while others need more time and space to refine and integrate the work. At the same time, the open-ended schedule might feel too loose for some people, who may need more structure for their daily practice.

It seems to me, as I review my library of perhaps thirty practice manuals of all shapes and sizes, that the more recent publications favor the open-ended kind of schedule. While I'm tempted to provide you with a couple of structured practice outlines, one for the slow lane and one for the fast, I feel it's best to take the open-ended route. Rather than try to prescribe fixed schedules for all the different students who read this guide—and I like to imagine that there will be a lot of you out there—I'll just offer some general practice guidelines and let you determine exactly how to manage your breathing affairs.

I've divided this schedule outline into four general practice levels, with levels 2 and 4 each having two parts. Refer to the index of practices whenever you need to find a specific exercise, posture, tool, support, or whatnot.

How Much Time

Before you go on to the practice levels, though, there's one question to consider: how much time are you willing to spend each day on your practice? Most people nowadays have very little spare time in their average day, and adding one more responsibility can seem like laying on that last straw that finally wrenches the camel's back and sends him off to the chiropractor. But it seems to me that, however busy you are during the day, somewhere in its 1,440 minutes there's a run of at least fifteen to twenty minutes available for this life-transforming practice of pranayama—after all, that's only a bit more than 1 percent of your day.

Anything less than fifteen minutes is really too little time to get much benefit from the practice, though on those days when any practice at all seems impossible, even five minutes is better than nothing. Naturally you could practice more than twenty minutes if you like, which means you're probably an unmarried, childless individual with a well-paying part-time job. Good for you.

Remember that, as with any other skill or art you're trying to acquire, the more time you dedicate to your practice, the more rapidly you'll advance and realize its benefits. As Patanjali recognized, the goal of yoga is very close to those who are vehement (samvega) in their practice and farther away from those who are only modest (mridu).

How to Find a Teacher

When you feel the time is right for personal instruction, there are several ways to find the perfect yoga teacher. Start by looking in your local Yellow Pages under "Yoga Instruction." Phone the nearby schools or individuals listed there and ask them to mail you a schedule of their classes and any other information they have that might be useful to a new student. *Yoga Journal,* the most widely read yoga magazine in this country, publishes an annual "Yoga Teachers Directory," which lists teachers (who pay a small fee for the listing) state by state. The magazine also has a teacher directory posted on its website at *www.yogajournal.com.* You could also ask your friends or associates at work to recommend a teacher or school. I'd be surprised if you didn't know someone, or know someone who knows someone, who takes a yoga class. Many athletic clubs also offer yoga classes to their members, so if you belong to a club, check its schedule.

Even though you may consider yourself to be in perfect shape, some yoga classes can be a real workout that will have you begging for mercy, so you'll probably want to start with a beginners' class. Most beginning classes are ongoing, which means that you'll be joining a more experienced group of students. If this seems intimidating, remember that just about everyone in the room, including the teacher, was a beginner once, too.

Once you've gathered all your information, talk to someone at each school or, if possible, talk to the teachers of any of the classes in which you're interested. Be sure to find out something about the school's approach first: some classes (like Ashtanga Vinyasa) are notoriously vigorous, while others (like Kripalu) are much milder. Be sure you have some idea of what you're getting into before you go, to avoid unpleasant surprises. You'll also want to know, if possible, the average size and length of the class, its cost, what kind of dress is recommended, and if the school provides you with a mat or blanket or if you need to bring your own.

If you have any physical problems or limitations, briefly describe them and see whether the teacher seems comfortable with the idea of working with you. You might ask about her training, certifications, and teaching experience. Next, if you're able to sample a few different teachers, try one or more classes with each one. Don't expect miracles. If nothing "happens" after the first class, don't be discouraged. Try again, or try another teacher or another school, until you find the right situation for you. Give yoga a fair chance.

Once you've settled on a teacher, it's best to study with that one person as much as possible, especially if you're working with a particular problem. This gives the teacher time to get to know you so that she can tailor postures and instructions to suit your needs.

Practice Level 1

Practice level 1 is a snap. Read through the introduction and the first part of this guide—that is, chapters 1 through 6. Buy yourself a blank notebook and write on the cover "MY PRANAYAMA JOUR-NAL," in big block letters, along with the date.

You might, before you do start your formal practice, write a short yoga autobiography in your journal. Why did you begin your practice of yoga? Just for the physical exercise? Or were there other reasons beyond this? What is yoga, anyway? Don't answer this question as you think the "experts" might; just write from your own experience. And ask yourself, Who am I? Does this question have any meaning to you? All of this will help you clarify your position at the very start of your trip into the country of the Self.

You'll also need to accumulate whatever props you think you'll want for your practice. But be reasonable and don't rush out and spend a fortune on props. Make or improvise, rather than buy, as many of your props as you can until you're sure, first, that you'll actually use them in practice and, second (and more important), that you intend to make pranayama a part of your daily routine.

> Total time through level 1: I estimate it will take you about a week to read the guide material and gather your journal and props—unless you're like me, in which case it will take closer to two weeks.

Practice Level 2

Practice level 2 has two parts. Part 1 generally covers chapters 7 and 8, then part 2 will take you from chapter 9 through chapter 12. You might also look at chapter 14 in Part Three of the guide. The asanas described in that chapter can be applied as warm-ups for Corpse, or you could wait to learn them until you begin formal pranayama in practice level 3.

Level 2: Part 1

Part 1 of this level begins by acquainting yourself with your Witness, who will be your constant companion for the rest of your voyage. Spend some time each day in Corpse doing nothing more than witnessing yourself, asking the question: Who am I?

Realistically it will take you a good while to cement this friendship, certainly more than a few weeks, but it's well worth the time and effort. Spend as much time as you can with your Witness during the day, watching yourself in all kinds of situations as you go about your business. It's easy enough to witness yourself when you're lying safe and warm and quiet in Corpse, but it's a considerably greater challenge when you're flying down the freeway and that so-and-so in front of you cuts into your lane without signaling.

Hand in hand with your Witness project, develop and refine your Corpse. Some students will already be familiar with Corpse from their asana classes and so won't need a lot of time to get comfortable in this posture. But if you're working with this asana as a novice, give yourself at least three weeks of consistent practice. Corpse is a valuable tool, not only in yoga practice but also anytime during the day that you feel you need to stop and smell the roses—early in the morning to get yourself primed for a busy day, in the afternoon after lunch, or to cool down just before bed.

Don't forget to work with your sensory body as well, both in Corpse and as you go about your business. The senses, like a barometer, respond to small moment-to-moment rises and falls in your internal pressures, signaling changes in your emotional weather. Experiment with the Six-Openings Seal.

> Time of daily practice: a minimum of fifteen to twenty minutes

> Total time through part 1 of level 2: for inexperienced Corpse practitioners, a minimum of three weeks to a month

Level 2: Part 2

Once you can lie comfortably in Corpse for ten to fifteen minutes, you can commence part 2 of this practice level with the mapping of your outer body and its inner space. Just as with befriending your Witness, mapping is a long process. But in Hatha-Yoga body knowledge always precedes and anchors self-knowledge. Draft a relatively clear chart of your body-self before venturing too far away from this home base. Without an adequate map, it's fairly easy to wander off the trail and get lost, especially if you don't have a live teacher around to keep you on course. If you're already an experienced asana student, mapping shouldn't take all that long, but beginners should give themselves a few weeks.

Once you have your map sketched out, learn as much as you can in the reclining position about the four qualities of your everyday breath. Be sure to witness these qualities in all kinds of situations. Find out, for example, what causes your time to speed up or slow down, what inevitably roughens your breath's texture, or how it happens that your space expands into the infinite or clams up tight. Come to a preliminary understanding of the surface breather and liberate as much of the authentic breather as you can before you try to change anything about your breathing behavior in unusual breathing. Repeat the mantra "Who is the breather?" to yourself throughout the day.

Then, after three weeks or so of everyday breathing, move on to the unusual-breathing exercises. They'll give you your first taste of purposeful control of your breathing rhythms. You can do one unusual breath each practice session or, if you have the time, work with two or more. But be sure to give them all an equal opportunity. Be alert, in fact, all through your practice for those exercises that you favor and those that, for whatever reasons, you don't like. Usually (though not always) the exercises that give you the most trouble are the ones with which you need to work the most. Spend at least a month with unusual breathing.

> Time of daily practice: a minimum of fifteen to twenty minutes
>
> Total time through part 2 of level 2: a minimum of two months
>
> Total time through level 2: a minimum of three months

Practice Level 3

Practice level 3 gets you into pranayama breathing proper. It generally covers chapters 13 through 15 in Part Three of the guide and chapters 17 through 19 in Part Four.

If you haven't already started working with the asanas in chapter

14, be sure to start now. Remember that asanas, while they have transformative value in and of themselves, have always been primarily a preparation for pranayama. If you don't have a regular asana practice, I urge you to either find a class or buy a book or video that will help you start one. I've listed my favorite yoga books and videos in the "Recommended Reading" section, though there's really no substitute for a living, breathing teacher.

The nine asanas in this guide are provided as simple warm-ups for your practice and helpers to free stuck areas in your groins, shoulders, or other parts of your body. Feel free to use other warm-up asanas you learn from your teacher, books, or videos.

After working and getting familiar with unusual breathing, you're ready to begin practicing the two foundation breaths in this guide, Conqueror and Against-the-Grain, in the reclining position. Learn the ajapa-mantra, hand mudras, nasal balance, and Skull Brightener immediately.

You can practice Conqueror alone for a while or, if you're comfortable with zigzag breathing, both Conqueror and Against-the-Grain. If, however, full Against-the-Grain creates problems, return to zigzag breathing for a while longer. Don't forget to extend and witness your breathing rests in preparation for retention.

In general, for both the reclining and sitting practices, work initially without ratio breathing for ten days to two weeks, then go into equal ratio pranayama. Once you're comfortable with equal ratio, learn unequal ratio pranayama and Lower Belly Lock. In both reclining and sitting, too, learn Skull Brightener right away, picking up its speed, intensity, and number of repetitions over several weeks.

For about the last two weeks of your time in this level, end each of your practice sessions with a few minutes of everyday breathing in Chair Seat. Learn as much as you can about the qualities of your breath in this new, vertical position. Be sure to have your chair and other props set up ahead of time, all ready to go when you finish your reclining breathing.

> Time for each breath: five to eight minutes
>
> Time of daily practice: twenty to twenty-five minutes
>
> Total time through level 3: a minimum of three months

Practice Level 4

Practice level 4 has two parts. Here you'll complete the work from chapters 16 and 20 in the guide.

Level 4: Part 1

Part 1 begins with your full transition to Chair Seat and sitting breathing. Not all students should start out with the same breathing practice, though. Some will need to repeat the work with unusual breathing, while others can jump right into the deep end with formal sitting pranayama.

How do you know which way to go? Be honest with yourself. If the transition from horizontal to vertical is causing you problems, then according to our lions, elephants, and tigers, you'll need to start cautiously with unusual breathing. If the problems persist, then it's possible you may have to return to the floor again for a week or two or three. Give yourself some time, then, with unusual breathing before you move along to formal pranayama.

But if the transition to chair sitting goes relatively smoothly, then you can start with unratioed Conqueror and Against-the-Grain, retracing the steps you took with these breaths through your reclining practice.

After a couple of weeks or so with these practices in Chair Seat, learn Net-Bearer Lock. Work on the lock itself at first; don't worry about actually retaining your breath. Needless to say, exercise extreme caution until you're sure that your neck isn't being tweaked. You might want to use a rolled-up washcloth or an elastic bandage as a chin support to relieve any strain. If this lock turns out to be a pain in the neck, though, stop immediately and seek the help of an experienced teacher.

Then, along with equal and unequal ratio breathing, begin to work with retention. Hold only for a count or two for the first week or so, then lengthen the time of the retention slowly with all due respect to the lions, elephants, and tigers. You might, for example, add one count each week until you reach the same count as your inhale. Practice at this count for a while before you venture out beyond the inhale count with retention.

Toward the end of your time in Chair Seat, begin to sit in a traditional seat at the end of each practice session. Unless you're already an experienced sitter, use your yoga wall for a back support. Experiment with the three seats described in this guide (you'll need to put a bolster between your back and the wall in Hero). Do this for at least two weeks with everyday breathing. Gradually lengthen the time you spend in your traditional seat for up to ten minutes.

> Time for each breath: a minimum of eight to ten minutes
>
> Time of daily practice: a minimum of twenty-five minutes
>
> Total time through part 1 of level 4: a minimum of two months

Level 4: Part 2

The second part of this practice level begins when you make your full transition to traditional sitting. By this time you're eight or nine months into your journey and should have a pretty good idea of how best to schedule your time. Your work in Chair Seat will supply you with the outline for your work in traditional sitting.

Develop and refine your traditional sitting practice step-by-step, without hurry or goal seeking. Learn to sit steadily and comfortably without a wall support. Slowly increase the time of your retention. Take one day each week and devote an hour-long practice session solely to pranayama.

Now that you're more confident of your breathing, be sure to experiment with your practice. This is certainly not the only pranayama guide available in the yoga marketplace. What do other teachers have to say about this practice, and what of value can they add to your work? Remember that no one teacher has all the answers.

> Time for each breath: a minimum of eight to ten minutes
>
> Time of daily practice: a minimum of twenty-five minutes
>
> Total time through part 2 of level 4: a minimum of three months
>
> Total time through level 4: a minimum of five months

Breathing with a Friend

Relationship . . . is the mirror in which you discover yourself. Without relationship you are not; to be is to be related; to be related is existence. You exist only in relationship; otherwise you do not exist, existence has no meaning. It is not because you think you are that you come into existence. You exist because you are related; and it is the lack of understanding of relationship that causes conflict.

—J. Krishnamurti, *The First and Last Freedom*

PRELIMINARY

It's often useful to have a partner around to help you with your yoga practice, whether you're working on your postures or your breathing. A partner is a kind of "living prop," though unlike an inanimate object, a partner can respond to your needs and regulate her adjustment, or she can answer questions and provide information, advice, and confirmation. The two partners together can then engage in a yoga dialogue, through which both can sharpen observational and verbal skills.

Partners must agree to communicate candidly, not only with words but also with touch and breath, and appreciate the other's strengths and weaknesses. In this way the partners develop not just new techniques for practice but more successful strategies for living with others as well.

Remember, though, that a partner can also be a distraction. Be sure to agree beforehand on what kind of partnership you both favor. You could decide to:

- Be completely silent and communicate only through touch, breath, gesture, or physical example.

- Use a bare minimum of words and say only what is necessary to inform, clarify, question, and so forth.

- Engage in a running commentary on the practice. The sole restriction would be that the communication concern only what's occurring in the practice.

How Do You Make an Adjustment?

Without some formal training in yoga teaching or other kind of body work, putting your hands on another person's gross body can be a little daunting. But the partner adjustments described in this appendix are fairly simple and shouldn't cause any discomfiture, especially if the partners know and trust one another—and are ready to have some fun and learn something about themselves.

Partner work is, like meditation, a form of awareness training. But formal meditation is commonly practiced in isolation, while in a partnership each member must stay aware of both self and other. This increases the partners' range of experience and perspective. What are some things you should know about adjusting?

There are several things to do even before you touch your partner. Always start by calling on your Witness, who will have the double duty of watching both your partner and yourself. Then ground your position, whether you're sitting or standing, calm your breath, and relax (and on cold days warm) your hands.

Now look carefully at your partner. As my favorite yogi, Yogi Berra, once said, "You can see a lot just by looking." Ask yourself objectively, What's going on here? Find your partner's midline to use as a plumb line for your assessment and adjustments. For the body as a whole, this line usually follows the line of the spine, but remember that each limb—an arm or a leg, for example—also has a midline. Finally, see if you can mimic your partner's posture—if not physically, then at least imaginatively. Try to find out what it feels like to actually be your partner, whether she's standing, sitting, or reclining.

Make yourself available to your partner. His needs and/or wants should take precedence (though you shouldn't lose yourself in the process). Since your purpose is to work for the other, just stay present and have no goal but to help. At the same time, be willing to share your experience with the other. Be what's called a fair witness. Avoid communicating your own expectations and/or tensions. If you relay some information, do it directly, in plain language, without hints about what to feel.

Make your adjustments within the partner's capacity; don't expect the impossible. There's a fine line between urging him to work to his limits and pushing him beyond these limits and causing distress or injury. When in doubt—you know what I'm going to say—play safe. While your adjustment may be focused on a particular area of the body, stay conscious of the wider implications and possibilities. Be prepared to expand your adjustment if your partner is agreeable. Stay with the adjustment until the end. Don't let go prematurely.

When You're Being Adjusted, How Do You Help the Partner with the Adjustment?

First, make sure your partner knows you're ready to be adjusted. Then don't be shy about asking for what you want: more or less pressure or weight, higher or lower touch, whatever. Remember that you are in charge of the process and that the adjustment should suit you, not the adjuster.

Similarly, answer questions from the partner honestly. Don't worry about being "demanding" or "critical." If the partner questions you about the accuracy or effectiveness of an adjustment, say it's not right if it isn't, ask for a change if you want it.

HOW IT HELPS

No matter how experienced or self-aware you are, no doubt there are a few lingering pockets of avidya somewhere on or in your body-mind. In pranayama a helper can encourage you to get in touch with those forgotten or unacknowledged parts of yourself, such as your back torso, during a mapping expedition or reaffirm your connection with places you've visited before; establish that elusive alignment in Corpse or other postures; or discover more about the surface and authentic breathers.

We'll be working specifically with three partner exercises in this appendix, though many more are possible. I'll clue you in to a few more of these possibilities in the "Going Further" sections. The three exercises are particularly useful for beginning breathers, for mapping the back torso, aligning the body in Corpse, and meeting the everyday breather with a partner.

Mapping the Back Torso

A partner is especially helpful on those mapping expeditions to the backcountry of the torso. Here's an exercise that's very popular in my breathing classes. The mapmaker should sit in a comfortable yoga seat. I prefer Hero (see chapter 16), but any traditional sitting asana or Chair Seat will do. The helper should then sit behind the mapmaker, also in a comfortable seat. Since the mapmaker mostly just sits for this exercise, the following instructions are directed at the helper unless otherwise noted.

PRACTICE

Gather any props needed by the mapmaker or yourself to make your chosen sitting positions comfortable. First, prepare yourself as described earlier. Then lay your hands on and spread them across the mapmaker's shoulders. At the same time hook your fingertips lightly under his clavicles. Firmly press down on the tops of the shoulders and pull them away from the base of the neck, and lift the clavicles lightly away from the top pairs of ribs. Ask the mapmaker to soften the area around his sternum and open the eyes of his heart. Continue with these actions for a minute or so.

Then slowly slide your hands down the back of the torso and spread your hands on the scapulas, fingers pointing up toward the head. Ask the mapmaker to pretend that, as you spread your palms over his scapulas, his scapulas are spreading under your palms.

Press the scapulas against the back ribs and, using that action as a trigger, ask the mapmaker to lift his heart. Then, without physically moving your hands, scrub the scapulas down the back toward the tailbone. Hold here for another minute or two.

Then slide your hands farther down the back, turning the fingers out as you go, into the hollow of the lower back. With the bases of your palms parallel to the line of the spine and your thumbs pointing up, spread the lumbar muscles away from the spine.

Now your hands are directly over the roots of the mapmaker's diaphragm (chapter 12). Help him initiate his inhales from these roots. Use your hands to monitor the movement of the breath in the lower back. Does one side move differently than the other? How? Describe what you feel to the mapmaker and encourage him, either verbally or through touch, to balance the movement of the two sides on both the inhales and the exhales. Spend anywhere from three to five minutes with this exercise.

Finally, slide your hands down on the sacrum. As you did with the scapulas, spread your palms over the bone and ask the mapmaker to do the same with the sacrum. Have him soften his lower belly and then press the sacrum into the back of the pelvis. Then, without physically moving your hands, scrub the sacrum down toward the tailbone. Hold for a minute or two. Finish by sliding your hands down along the coccyx and lengthening it into the floor.

GOING FURTHER

The roots of the diaphragm is not the only solo exercise from the guide that you can do with a partner. Your partner can help you contact the floating ribs, outline the rim of the diaphragm, open the eyes of the heart, find the root of the neck, or create the Lower Belly Lock.

Aligning the Physical Body in Corpse

As I mentioned in the guide, it's very difficult at first to secure the right alignment for Corpse on our own, since our habitual misalignments are so ingrained. A partner can help you get the feel of alignment in Corpse so that you can re-create it in the posture later, by yourself.

The partner doing Corpse should lie either with her legs straight or with her knees supported on a round bolster. Since the Corpse mostly just lies there like, well, a corpse, the following instructions are directed at the helper unless otherwise noted.

PRACTICE: FEET

Gather whatever the Corpse needs to make himself comfortable. Look at the angles the two feet make relative to a line drawn between them perpendicular to the floor. The feet should angle evenly away from the perpendicular, but often one foot is more upright than the other. Usually this indicates some tightness in the same-side hip. Sometimes both feet are pretty vertical, and you can bet that there's some stickiness in both hips.

Slide your hands under the Corpse's heels and cradle them. Then gently rock his two legs back and forth, like a pair of windshield wipers, for thirty seconds to a minute. Make sure the pivot points for this rocking movement are in the hip joints, not in the knees or ankles. This should help to soften the tightness in her hips. Lay the feet back down lightly on the floor. Look again at their angles. Any better?

PRACTICE: PELVIS

Then look at the pair of significant landmarks on the front of the pelvis, the hip points, and draw a line between them. Is this line parallel to the floor? Often it will be tilted to one side or the other, indicating that the back of the pelvis isn't resting evenly on the floor. Straddle the Corpse's legs, bend forward, and press the bases of your palms lightly against his hip points. Rock them gently back and forth, pushing down first on one side, then the other. Recheck your adjustment. Any better?

Look at the hip-point line again and draw a companion line across the top of the shoulders. Are these two lines parallel to each other? You'll frequently see that they angle toward each other on one side, shortening that side of the torso relative to the other. Slide your hand under the short-side hip and pull it gently downward, lengthening the shorter side.

PRACTICE: SHOULDERS

Look at the shoulders. You'll often see that the shoulders are hunched toward the ears and pinched across the upper chest. Now straddle the Corpse's torso. Bend over, rest your left hand on the front of the left shoulder, and slide your right hand below the left shoulder, spreading your palm under the scapula. Draw the scapula down away from the ear and out away from the spine; at the same time, gently press your left hand against the head of the upper arm bone (humerus). Broaden the clavicles away from the sternum. Repeat on the right side.

Again, look at the line of the shoulders. Is it broader now, and are the tops of the shoulders equidistant from the ears? Make any small adjustments you think are necessary.

PRACTICE: ARMS AND HANDS

Just as with the heels, the backs of the hands should rest evenly on the floor, as close as possible to the knuckles of the index fingers. Often, though, you'll see an imbalance in the hands, one resting on the middle-finger knuckle, for example, the other closer to the pinky.

As you continue to straddle the Corpse's torso in a forward bend, press the bases of your thumbs against the bases of the his thumbs. Encourage him to further soften the shoulders and relax the roots of the thumbs, deep in the hands and forearms.

PRACTICE: NECK AND HEAD

Finally, look at the neck and head. The base of the skull will frequently be dragged down on the back of the neck, jutting the chin sharply up toward the ceiling. Bend over and slide your hands gently below the base of the skull. Lift it away from the back of the neck, bringing the chin approximately perpendicular to the floor. Usually a head like this will need some support under it, such as a folded blanket, to raise it off the floor.

As you did with the hip points, draw a line between the eyes. Is this line parallel to the floor? Often it's tilted over to one side, indicating that the Corpse's head isn't resting evenly on the floor. So adjust the head into a neutral position by rotating it in one direction or the other.

A partner can make similar adjustments when you're in your bolster-supported reclining pranayama position or sitting either in Chair Seat or on the floor.

Meeting the Everyday Breather with a Partner

In chapter 11 we worked to clarify the qualities of the everyday breather using our hands. Sometimes it's nice to just kick back and breathe and let someone else do all the hard hand work. That way we can focus on just breathing and get someone else's input about that breathing in the bargain.

The partner doing the breathing should lie in Corpse, either with his legs straight or with his knees supported on a round bolster. Since the breather's only responsibility is to breathe, the following instructions are directed to the helper unless otherwise noted.

PRACTICE

Use whatever props the breather needs to make himself comfortable. Straddle the breather and lean forward, bending your knees. Lay and spread your hands on the breather's front ribs, below the line of the nipples, fingers pointing to the sides. At first just let the breather feel your palms resting on his ribs. Then have him begin to breathe into your hands.

Witness the movement of your hands for a few minutes. What do you feel? It probably won't come as a surprise that your hands aren't moving evenly or equally. One hand—the right, for example—will be expanding more quickly than the left on the inhale, then lagging behind on the exhale. Or the hands will move in fits and starts, indicating something about the breath's texture. Just as you did with your body when assessing the mapmaker in the earlier exercise, try to mimic the breather's breath with your own.

In a soft voice describe what you're experiencing to the breather. Ask him to make whatever adjustments you feel are needed. Encourage the breather to expand and contract the rib case as smoothly and evenly as possible. Continue for a few minutes, then slide your hands together and lift them off the breather.

GOING FURTHER

The helper can also help the breather do such things as breathe into the eyes of the heart, find the rim of the diaphragm, descend the skin of the forehead, or work with the reclining version of the Lower Belly Lock.

Yoga Props

Nasal Wash

Narial Nasal Cup
Essential Products Alliance
P.O. Box 1003
Versailles, KY 40383
Phone: (800) 817-8740

Yoga Props

At One Yoga
10050 N. Scottsdale Rd., #115
Scottsdale, AZ 85253
Phone: (877) AT-1-YOGA
Web site: www.atoneyoga.com

Bheka Yoga Supplies
258 A St., Unit 6B
Ashland, OR 97520
Phone: (800) 366-4541

Fish Crane Yoga Props
Phone: (800) 959-6116

Hugger-Mugger Yoga Products
3937 S. 500 W.
Salt Lake City, UT 84123
Phone: (800) 473-4888
Web site: www.huggermugger.com

Kripalu Yogawear
P.O. Box 793
Lenox, MA 01240
Phone: (888) 399-1332
Web site: www.kripalu.org

Manduka Matsource
P.O. Box 14812
San Luis Obispo, CA 93406
Phone: (805) 544-9642
Web site: www.yogacentre.com

Tools for Yoga Prop Shop
2 Green Village Rd.
Madison, NJ 07940
Phone: (888) 678-9642
Web site: www.toolsforyoga.net

Unity Woods Beyondananda Boutique
4853 Cordell Ave. PH9
Bethesda, MD 20814
Phone: (301) 656-7792
Web site: www.unitywoods.com

Yoga Accessories
P.O. Box 13976
New Bern, NC 28561
Phone: (800) 990-9642
Web site: www.yogaaccessories.com

Yoga Props
3055-J Twenty-third St.
San Francisco, CA 94110
Phone: (888) 856-YOGA
Web site: www.yogaprops.net

Yogamats
P.O. Box 885044
San Francisco, CA 94188
Phone: (800) 720-YOGA
Web site: www.ecomall.com/biz/
yoga.htm

YogaPro
Phone: (800) 488-8414
Web site: www.yogapro.com

NOTES

INTRODUCTION Lions, Elephants, Tigers

1. Alain Danielou, *The Gods of India: Hindu Polytheism* (New York: Inner Traditions, 1985), p. 152.

2. Heinrich Zimmer, *Myths and Symbols in Indian Art and Civilization,* Bollingen Series, vol. 6, ed. Joseph Campbell (Princeton, N.J.: Princeton University Press, 1946), p. 13.

3. Svatmarama, *Hatha-Yoga-Pradipika,* with a commentary by Swami Muktibodhananda Saraswati (Munger, Bihar, India: Bihar School of Yoga, 1985), p. 506.

4. Ibid., p. 508.

5. *Shiva-Samhita,* trans. Rai Bahadur Srisa Chandra Vasu (New Delhi: Sri Satguru Publications, 1990), p. 35.

CHAPTER 1 The Yoga of Breathing

1. *The Thirteen Principal Upanishads,* trans. Robert Ernest Hume (London: Oxford University Press, 1931), pp. 351–52.

2. Unless otherwise noted, all translations of Patanjali in this guide are from *The Yoga-Sutra of Patanjali,* trans. Georg Feuerstein (Rochester, Vt.: Inner Traditions, 1979). Numbers in parentheses following each quote indicate its chapter and sutra number.

3. James Carse, *Finite and Infinite Games* (New York: Ballantine, 1986), p. 19.

4. Lama Anagarika Govinda, *Foundations of Tibetan Mysticism* (New Delhi: B.I. Publications, 1977), pp. 152–53.

5. *The Thirteen Principal Upanishads,* trans. Robert Ernest Hume (London: Oxford University Press, 1931), p. 95.

6. Ibid., pp. 307, 328.

CHAPTER 2 Shining Forth

1. Lama Anagarika Govinda, *Foundations of Tibetan Mysticism* (New Delhi: B.I. Publications, 1977), p. 154.

2. *The Bhagavad-Gita,* trans. R. C. Zaehner (London: Oxford University Press, 1969), p. 216.

3. Sri Aurobindo, *The Synthesis of Yoga* (Pondicherry, India: Sri Aurobindo Ashram, 1970), p. 205.

4. Heinrich Zimmer, *The Philosophies of India,* Bollingen Series, vol. 26, ed. Joseph Campbell (Princeton, N.J.: Princeton University Press, 1951), p. 298.

5. B. K. S. Iyengar, *Light on the Yoga-Sutras of Patanjali* (San Francisco: Aquarian Press, 1993), p. 30.

6. Bernard Bouanchaud, *The Essence of Yoga: Reflections on the Yoga-Sutras of Patanjali* (Portland, Oreg.: Rudra Press, 1997), p. 140.

7. Svatmarama, *Hatha-Yoga-Pradipika,* with a commentary by Swami Muktibodhananda Saraswati (Munger, Bihar, India: Bihar School of Yoga, 1985), p. 506.

8. *Thirteen Principal Upanishads,* trans. Robert Ernest Hume (London: Oxford University Press, 1931), p. 398.

9. John Woodroffe, *Shakti and Shiva* (New York: Dover, 1978), p. 685.

10. *Thirteen Principal Upanishads,* trans. Robert Ernest Hume (London: Oxford University Press, 1931), p. 267.

11. Ken Wilber, "Are the Chakras Real?" in *Kundalini: Evolution and Enlightenment,* ed. John White (New York: Paragon, 1990), p. 128.

12. Svatmarama, *Hatha-Yoga-Pradipika,* with a commentary by Swami Muktibodhananda Saraswati (Munger, Bihar, India: Bihar School of Yoga, 1985), p. 203.

13. Ibid., p. 134.

CHAPTER 3   Obstacles and Helpers

1. *Shiva-Samhita,* trans. Rai Bahadur Srisa Chandra Vasu (New Delhi: Sri Satguru Publications, 1990), p. 31.

2. Shankara, *Crest-Jewel of Discrimination,* trans. with an introduction by Swami Prabhavananda and Christopher Isherwood (New York: New American Library, 1947), p. 38.

3. *The Collected Works of Ramana Maharshi,* ed. Arthur Osborne (New York: Samuel Weiser, 1970), p. 39.

4. *Shiva-Samhita,* trans. Rai Bahadur Srisa Chandra Vasu (New Delhi: Sri Satguru Publications, 1990), p. 26.

5. *The Concise Yoga Vasishtha,* trans. Swami Venkatesananda (Albany: State University of New York Press, 1984), p. 35.

6. *The Yoga Philosophy of Patanjali,* trans. with a commentary by Swami Hariharananda Aranaya (Albany: State University of New York Press, 1983), p. 71.

7. *Shiva-Samhita,* trans. Rai Bahadur Srisa Chandra Vasu (New Delhi: Sri Satguru Publications, 1990), p. 43.

CHAPTER 4 Props

1. *Gheranda-Samhita,* trans. Rai Bahadur Chandra Vasu (New Delhi: Sri Satguru Publications, 1979), pp. 27–28.

CHAPTER 5 Practice Tips

1. *Yoga-Sutras of Patanjali, vol. 1, Samadhi-pada,* trans. with a commentary by Pandit Usarbudh Arya (Honesdale, Pa.: Himalayan International Institute of Yoga Science and Philosophy of the U.S.A., 1986), p. 37.

CHAPTER 7 The Witness

1. Sri Aurobindo, *The Synthesis of Yoga* (Pondicherry, India: Sri Aurobindo Ashram, 1970), p. 226.
2. Paul Deussen, *The System of the Vedanta,* trans. Charles Johnston (New York: Dover, 1973), p. 324.

CHAPTER 8 Corpse: Introduction to Shavasana

1. *The Bhagavad-Gita,* trans. R. C. Zaehner (London: Oxford University Press, 1969), p. 133.
2. Svatmarama, *Hatha-Yoga-Pradipika,* with a commentary by Swami Muktibodhananda Saraswati (Munger, Bihar, India: Bihar School of Yoga, 1985), p. 86.

CHAPTER 10 Quieting the Sense Organs in Corpse

1. *Yoga-Sutras of Patanjali, vol. 1, Samadhi-pada,* trans. with a commentary by Pandit Usarbudh Arya (Honesdale, Pa.: Himalayan International Institute of Yoga Science and Philosophy of the U.S.A., 1986), p. 245.
2. *Pure Yoga,* trans. Yogi Pranavananda (Delhi: Motilal Banarsidass, 1992), p. 75.

CHAPTER 11 Qualities of the Breath: Time, Texture, Space, and Rest

1. *The Yoga-System of Patanjali,* trans. James H. Woods, Harvard Oriental Series, vol. 17 (Cambridge, Mass.: Harvard University Press, 1927), p. 194.
2. *Svatmarama, Hatha-Yoga-Pradipika,* with a commentary by Swami Muktibodhananda Saraswati (Munger, Bihar, India: Bihar School of Yoga, 1985), p. 134.

CHAPTER 12 Unusual Breathing

1. Mabel Todd, *The Thinking Body* (New York: Dance Horizons, 1937), p. 229.

CHAPTER 14   Posture

1. *The Bhagavad-Gita,* trans. R. C. Zaehner (London: Oxford University Press, 1969), p. 224.
2. *The Yoga-Sutra of Patanjali,* trans. Georg Feuerstein (Rochester, Vt.: Inner Traditions, 1979), pp. 90–91.
3. *Gheranda-Samhita,* trans. Rai Bahadur Chandra Vasu (New Delhi: Sri Satguru Publications, 1979), p. 2.

CHAPTER 16   Traditional Seats

1. Svatmarama, *Hatha-Yoga-Pradipika,* with a commentary by Swami Muktibodhananda Saraswati (Munger, Bihar, India: Bihar School of Yoga, 1985), pp. 97–98.

CHAPTER 17   Tools

1. Heinrich Zimmer, *Myths and Symbols in Indian Art and Civilization,* Bollingen Series, vol. 6, ed. Joseph Campbell (Princeton, N.J.: Princeton University Press, 1946), p. 48.
2. Ibid., pp. 48–49.
3. Ibid., p. 50.
4. Svatmarama, *Hatha-Yoga-Pradipika,* with a commentary by Swami Muktibodhananda Saraswati (Munger, Bihar, India: Bihar School of Yoga, 1985), p. 211.

CHAPTER 18   Conqueror's Breath

1. Alphonse Goettmann, *Dialogue on the Path of Initiation: An Introduction to the Life and Thought of Karlfried Graf Durckheim,* trans. Theodore Nottingham and Rebecca Nottingham (New York: Globe Press, 1991), p. 94.
2. *The Yoga of Delight, Wonder, and Astonishment,* trans. of the *Vijnana-Bhairava* by Jaideva Singh (Albany: State University of New York Press, 1991), p. 47.
3. Alphonse Goettmann, *Dialogue on the Path of Initiation: An Introduction to the Life and Thought of Karlfried Graf Durckheim,* trans. Theodore Nottingham and Rebecca Nottingham (New York: Globe Press, 1991), p. 96.
4. Quoted in Lilian Silburn, *Kundalini: The Energy of the Depths,* trans. Jacques Gontier (Albany: State University of New York Press, 1988), p. 110.

CHAPTER 20   Locks and Retention

1. Svatmarama, Hatha-Yoga-Pradipika, with a commentary by Swami Muktibodhananda Saraswati (Munger, Bihar, India: Bihar School of Yoga, 1985), p. 211.

2. Theos Bernard, *Hatha Yoga* (New York: Samuel Weiser, 1968), p. 51.

3. Alain Danielou, *Yoga: Mastering the Secrets of Matter and the Universe* (Rochester, Vt.: Inner Traditions, 1991), p. 53.

4. Theos Bernard, *Hatha Yoga* (New York: Samuel Weiser, 1968), p. 70.

5. *The Bhagavad-Gita,* trans. by Barbara Stoler Miller (New York: Bantam Books, 1986), p. 35.

GLOSSARY

Abhinivesha Will to live, tenacity; one of the five causes of affliction. *See also* klesha.

Abhyasa Practice, repeated or permanent exercise, discipline.

Adhikara Qualification, entitled to, fit for.

Ajna-chakra Wheel of command; the sixth of seven major energy centers in the human subtle body, located in the space between the eyebrows.

Amrita Immortal, imperishable; the nectar of immortality, sometimes said to drip from the base of the brain.

Ananta Infinite, endless, boundless, eternal; sometimes used to refer to the thousand-headed snake, an emblem of eternity, also called Remainder or Residue (shesha).

Antaraya Obstacle, any impediment to the ultimate goals of yoga. There are nine in classical yoga: sickness (vyadhi), languor (styana), doubt (samshaya), heedlessness (pramada), sloth (alasya), dissipation (avirati), false vision (bhranti-darshana), nonattainment of yogic stages (alabdha-bhumikatva), and instability in these stages (anavasthitatva).

Apana-vayu Downward wind, one of the five vital currents, responsible for elimination.

Apavarga Completion, emancipation, beatitude.

Asana Seat, derived from as, "to sit quietly, abide, remain, continue."

Ashta-anga-yoga Eight-limb yoga, the classical practice of yama, niyama, asana, pranayama, pratyahara, dharana, dhyana, and samadhi.

Asmita I-am-ness, from asmi, "I am."

Atman The self, variously derived from an, "to breathe"; at, "to move"; and va, "to blow."

Avidya Not-knowing, unwise, unlearned, spiritual ignorance.

Bandha Lock or bond.

Bhakti Devotion.

Bhavanatas Projection, the name given collectively to four positive states of consciousness: friendliness (maitri), compassion (karuna), gladness (mudita), and equanimity (upeksha).

Brahma-dvara Brahma gate or entrance, the inlet of the sushumna-nadi at the base of the spine.

Brahma-randhra Brahma opening, the outlet of the sushumna-nadi at the crown of the head.

Buddhi The higher mind, from budh, "to be awake."

Cakra Energy center or wheel; traditionally there are seven of these wheels located in the sushumna-nadi.

Cit Transcendental consciousness; literally, to perceive, attend to.

Citta Human consciousness.

Dharana Concentration, the sixth of eight limbs of classical yoga.

Dhyana Meditation, the seventh of eight limbs of classical yoga.

Duhkha Variously translated as sorrow, suffering, pain, misery.

Dvadasha-anta Literally, the "end of twelve"; energetic centers similar to cakras, some of which are located outside the body.

Dvesha Aversion, one of the five causes of affliction (klesha) in classical yoga.

Guna Strand, quality; traditionally there are three gunas: tamas, rajas, and sattva.

Ida-nadi The comfort channel, one of the three main nadis in the subtle body, situated to the left of sushumna-nadi.

Indriya Belonging to Indra; refers to the eleven sense organs (according to classical yoga), including five cognitive senses (jnana-indriya)—eyes, ears, nose, tongue, skin; five conative senses (karma-indriya)—hands, feet, voice, anus, genitals; and the lower mind (manas).

Ishvara The Lord of classical yoga.

Japa Recitation or muttering of prayers or mantras.

Jiva-atman The living or embodied self.

Jivan-mukti Living or embodied liberation.

Jnana Higher wisdom.

Kaivalya Aloneness, detachment of the self from all nature and from transmigration, the ultimate state of liberation in classical yoga.

Kanda Egg-shaped bulb, the root of all the energy channels (nadi), usually located at the base of the spine.

Karma Action.

Kevala-kumbhaka Absolute retention, the consummation of the practice of retention (kumbhaka).

Klesha Cause of affliction, pain. Five are listed by Patanjali: the root cause, spiritual ignorance (avidya), along with I-am-ness (asmita), attachment (raga), aversion (dvesha), and the will to live (abhinivesha).

Kumbha Pot, used to describe the human torso.

Kumbhaka Potlike, the practice of retention in general.

Manas The lower mind.

Mantra Hymn or prayer.

Meru-danda The staff of Meru, another name for the human spine, which is compared to Mount Meru, the mythic mountain at the center of the Hindu universe.

Moksha Liberation or emancipation.

Mudra Seal, generally a muscular contraction of the body or a symbolic arrangement of the hands.

Mukhya-prana First prana, a name for cosmic prana as differentiated from individual prana. *See also* vasti-prana.

Mumukshutva Eagerness to be free, striving after liberation.

Nada The subtle inner sound.

Nadi A vital energy channel of the subtle body.

Nadi-cakra The entire network or wheel of the vital energy channels (nadi).

Nirodha Restraint, control.

Niyama Restraint, the second limb of the eight-limb discipline, consisting of purity (shauca), contentment (samtosha), asceticism (tapas), scriptural study (svadhyaya), and devotion to the Lord (ishvara-pranidhana).

Pari-karman The yogic helpers.

Pingala-nadi The tawny channel, one of the three main channels in the subtle body, situated to the right of sushumna-nadi.

Prakriti Matter or nature.

Prana Vital energy.

Prana-vayu Forward wind, one of the five vital currents, responsible for appropriation.

Pratyahara Self-restraint, the fifth limb of the eight-limb discipline.

Purusha The self.

Raga Attachment, one of the five causes of affliction (klesha).

Rajas Energy, one of the three gunas.

Raja-Yoga Royal yoga, another name for the classical yoga of Patanjali.

Sahasrara-cakra The energy wheel at the crown of the head.

Sakshin The Witness, often used to refer to the self.

Samadhi Literally, putting together, the eighth limb of the eight-limb discipline.

Samana-vayu Middle wind, one of the five vital currents, responsible for assimilation; the fire in the belly.

Samasti-prana Whole prana, a name for cosmic prana as differentiated from individual prana (vasti-prana).

Samatva Evenness, balance.

Samtosha Contentment, one of the five niyamas.

Sattva Beingness, one of the three gunas.

Siddhi Accomplishment, fulfillment, complete attainment.

Sukha Easy, pleasant.

Sushumna-nadi The most gracious channel, the central channel of the subtle network of nadis.

Svadhyaya Scriptural study, listed as both one of the five niyamas and three practices of Patanjali's yoga of action (kriya-yoga).

Tamas Darkness, inertia, one of the three gunas.

Udana-vayu Upward wind, one of the five vital currents, responsible for expression.

Vairagya Dispassion, freedom from worldly desires; literally, growing pale.

Vasti-prana Individual prana, as differentiated from cosmic prana. *See also* mukhya-prana, samasti-prana.

Vikshepa Distraction, confusion, the four attendants of the classical obstacles (antaraya): suffering or pain (duhkha), depression or melancholy (daurmanasya), physical restlessness (angam-ejatva), and disturbed breathing.

Viveka Discernment, discrimination.

Vritti Fluctuation, a movement in consciousness (citta).

Vyana-vayu Circulating wind, one of the five vital currents, responsible for circulation.

Yama Restraint, ethical observance, the first limb of the eight-limb discipline, consisting of nonharming (ahimsa), truthfulness (satya), non-stealing (asteya), sexual restraint (brahmacarya), and greedlessness (aparigraha).

RECOMMENDED READING

ASANA INSTRUCTION

Couch, Jean. *The Runner's Yoga Book*. Berkeley, Calif.: Rodmell Press, 1990.

Iyengar, B. K. S. *Light on Yoga*. New York: Schocken, 1979.

Lassater, Judith, Ph.D., P.T. *Relax and Renew*. Berkeley, Calif.: Rodmell Press, 1995.

Schiffmann, Erich. *Yoga: The Spirit and Practice of Moving into Stillness*. New York: Pocket Books, 1996.

BASIC ANATOMY

Calais-Germain, Blandine. *Anatomy of Movement*. Seattle: Eastland Press, 1993.

Calais-Germain, Blandine, and Andrée Lamotte. *Anatomy of Movement Exercises*. Seattle: Eastland Press, 1996.

Olsen, Andrea, in collaboration with Caryn McHose. *BodyStories: A Guide to Experiential Anatomy*. Barrytown, N.Y.: Station Hill Press, 1991.

Todd, Mabel. *The Thinking Body*. New York: Dance Horizons, 1937.

CLASSICAL YOGA: TRANSLATIONS OF THE YOGA-SUTRA

Bouanchaud, Bernard. *The Essence of Yoga: Reflections on the Yoga-Sutra of Patanjali*. Portland, Oreg.: Rudra Press, 1997.

Feuerstein, Georg. *The Yoga-Sutra of Patanjali*. Rochester, Vt.: Inner Traditions, 1989.

Iyengar, B. K. S. *Light on the Yoga-Sutras of Patanjali*. San Francisco: Aquarian Press, 1993.

Miller, Barbara Stoler. *Yoga: Discipline of Freedom: The Yoga-Sutra Attributed to Patanjali*. Berkeley, Calif.: University of California Press, 1996.

HATHA-YOGA

Svatmarama. *Hatha-Yoga-Pradipika*. Commentary by Swami Vishnu-devananda. New York: Om Lotus Publications, 1987.

GENERAL BREATHING

Farhi, Donna. *The Breathing Book.* New York: Henry Holt, 1996.
Hendricks, Gay, Ph.D. *Conscious Breathing.* New York: Bantam, 1995.

GENERAL YOGA

Desikachar, T. K. V. *The Heart of Yoga.* Rochester, Vt.: Inner Traditions, 1995.
Feuerstein, Georg. *The Shambhala Guide to Yoga.* Boston: Shambhala Publications, 1996.
———. *Teachings of Yoga.* Boston: Shambhala Publications, 1997.
Graf von Durckheim, Karlfried. *The Way of Transformation.* London: Unwin, 1971.
Iyengar, B. K. S. *The Tree of Yoga.* Boston: Shambhala Publications, 1989.

JOURNAL WRITING AND SPIRITUAL JOURNAL-GUIDES

Gendlin, Eugene. *Focusing.* New York: Bantam, 1978.
Merrell-Wolff, Franklin. *Pathways through to Space.* New York: Julian Press, 1973.
Progoff, Ira. *At a Journal Workshop.* New York: Dialogue House, 1975.
———. *The Practice of Process Meditation.* New York: Dialogue House, 1980.
Tweedie, Irina. *The Chasm of Fire.* The Old Brewery, Tisbury, Wiltshire, U.K.: Element Books, 1979.

KUNDALINI

Radha, Swami Sivananda. *Kundalini Yoga for the West.* Boulder, Colo.: Shambhala Publications, 1981.
White, John, ed. Kundalini, *Evolution and Enlightenment.* New York: Paragon House, 1990.

THE WITNESS AND CONSCIOUSNESS

Bentov, Itzhak. *Stalking the Wild Pendulum.* New York: Dutton, 1977.
Osborne, Arthur, ed. *The Collected Works of Ramana Maharshi.* New York: Samuel Weiser, 1972.
Wilber, Ken. *The Spectrum of Consciousness.* Wheaton, Ill.: Theosophical Publishing House, 1977.

PRANAYAMA INSTRUCTION

Iyengar, B. K. S. *Light on Pranayama.* New York: Crossroad, 1981.
Rama, Swami; Rudolph Ballentine, M.D.; and Alan Hymes, M.D. *Science of Breath.* Honesdale, Pa.: Himalayan International Institute of Yoga Science and Philosophy, 1979.

INDEX OF PRACTICES